D0981954

Fast
BURN!

Also by Ian K. Smith, M.D.

Mind over Weight

Clean & Lean

The Clean 20

Blast the Sugar Out!

The SHRED Power Cleanse

The SHRED Diet Cookbook

SUPER SHRED

SHRED

The Truth About Men

Eat

Happy

The 4 Day Diet

Extreme Fat Smash Diet

The Fat Smash Diet

The Take-Control Diet

Dr. Ian Smith's Guide to Medical Websites

Novels

The Ancient Nine

The Blackbird Papers

The Unspoken

Fast
BURN!

THE POWER OF NEGATIVE ENERGY BALANCE

Ian K. Smith, M.D.

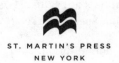

ST. MARTIN'S PRESS
NEW YORK

First published in the United States by St. Martin's Press, an imprint of St. Martin's Publishing Group

www.stmartins.com

Library of Congress Cataloging-in-Publication Data

Names: Smith, Ian, 1969– author.
Title: Fast burn! : the power of negative energy balance / Ian K. Smith, M.D.
Description: First edition. | New York : St. Martin's Press, 2021. | Includes index.
Identifiers: LCCN 2020048576 | ISBN 9781250271587 (hardcover) | ISBN 9781250271594 (ebook)
Subjects: LCSH: Reducing diets. | Reducing diets—Recipes. | Nutrition. | Exercise.
Classification: LCC RM222.2 .S62217 2021 | DDC 613.2/5—dc23
LC record available at https://lccn.loc.gov/2020048576

Our books may be purchased in bulk for promotional, educational, or business use. Please contact your local bookseller or the Macmillan Corporate and Premium Sales Department at 1-800-221-7945, extension 5442, or by email at MacmillanSpecialMarkets@macmillan.com.

First Edition: 2021

10 9 8 7 6 5 4 3 2 1

To my beautiful, talented, smart, creative, athletic nieces Storie and Sonix. The two of you are part of our family's future. Carry the torch well and with pride. I love you.

Contents

CONTENTS

A Note from the Author

Throughout my career, I have learned a lot more than I have taught. One of the biggest lessons that I've learned has been that regardless of how great a diet plan might be or how effective it has been for a large number of people, there's no one diet plan that fits everyone. All of us lose weight differently, and we respond differently to the methods and strategies that are designed to help us get rid of those unwanted pounds.

Over the last year I received a significant amount of feedback from people who come from all walks of life. They had experienced varying degrees of weight loss success following a broad array of programs. If I had to rank the queries by frequency, the two most common questions had to do with the most effective strategies to burn fat and how these results could be achieved quickly. I decided to go back to school and look more intensely at the physiology of fat—how it grows and how it shrinks. I wanted to reacquaint myself with the relationship between the fat we eat and the fat that appears underneath our skin, around our organs, and other highly visible areas we would prefer it not exist. I then looked at some of the latest research to see if it was possible to better attack our body fat and to do so in a way that wouldn't make this mission take the better part of a year to accomplish.

FAST BURN is the accumulation—the culmination—of what I discovered. I've taken what can be complicated science and distilled it into a nine-week plan that offers you a chance to reach your goals (presuming they're reasonable) in a relatively accelerated time frame safely and without going to extremes. I've provided as much flexibility as I can, but there is still a need to have some structure so that the basic tenets of weight loss remain intact and help deliver the results many are so desperate to achieve. It's very possible that after completing these nine weeks, you decide to adopt this style of eating for the rest of your life. It's not that you will be obligated to follow a specific regimen, but you will take those aspects of the program that worked best for you and make them a permanent routine in your eating style. You will experience real change over these nine weeks, changes that I hope will not be temporary, but rather sustainable and long term. If you believe in yourself first, then believe in the plan, and then put in the work, you will find that at the end of nine weeks, you are a different person physically and mentally than you were when you began the journey. There's one tenet of all diet plans that continues to stand the test of time. You get out of it what you put into it. Work hard. Don't be too hard on yourself. And have fun. **FAST BURN** is a plan built in a way that you can follow for life!

Ian K. Smith, M.D.
April 2021

Acknowledgments

On the publication of this, my twentieth book, there are many people who have ardently supported my work. Thousands of people have joined my online Facebook challenges and my admins Beverly, Felicia, Sandra, and Rosemary have helped guide them. They tested various portions of the program and reported their results and gave me suggestions to enhance the plan and improve it to what you see today. Thanks to my long-time editor Elizabeth Beier who knows my cadence and helps my ideas and voice reach new heights. Hannah Phillips, thanks for keeping the trains on the track and running on time. I appreciate you. Thanks to my good friend and terrible golfer, Steve Cohen, the reason why I found St. Martin's Press so many years ago and one of the big reasons why I still continue to publish there. John Karle, Brant Janeway, Erica Martirano, Laura Clark, Jen Enderlin, and the rest of the St. Martin's team—you guys rock and work hard to make my words sing. John Sargent, thanks for being a great Big Boss and protecting and nourishing and supporting all of those at Macmillan who were lucky to work with you. If only other CEOs could duplicate even some of what you've done and how you've comported yourself over all these years with grace, dignity, and humanity. I look forward to your next chapter. You have made publishing a lot of fun for me! And, of course, my personal team that gives me all the reasons in the world to do what I do and to be happy while doing it: Tristé, Dashiell, and Declan. You guys know where my heart lives. I love you!

Fast
BURN!

1

The Fat Truth

THERE'S A REALLY GOOD REASON WHY WE HAVE A LOVE-HATE relationship with fat. We love the way it tastes, but we despise what too much of it can do to the appearance of our body. We enjoy that fatty piece of ribeye and those French fries and creamy alfredo sauce, because the fat we consume tastes good and triggers the release of the neurotransmitter dopamine in our brains that brings us a sense of satisfaction and pleasure. But on the other side of the equation, fat that we consume, as well as excess calories that we don't burn off, increase the amount of body fat that is stored under our skin and around our vital organs. Excess fat and calories inconveniently find their way into our abdomen, causing an unwanted protrusion, or on the back of our arms or underneath our chins. We have a schizophrenic relationship with fat—we want it, but then we don't want it. You're reading this book because you want to know how to get rid of all that unwanted fat that's making your clothes fit too tight or has you contemplating how different you might look after a session of liposuction, or maybe it's causing your insulin hormone to not function well, and thus your blood sugars are high. All of these scenarios and others prompt us to want significant change, but before we talk about burning the fat, let's get a quick understanding of what it is and why we actually need it—at least some of it, in appropriate amounts.

What Is Fat?

Fat: you know it when you see it. Whether it's the rim around a pork chop or the streaks running through a steak or the dimpling you can see under a tight dress—fat is everywhere. Fat is considered one of the three macronutrients—nutrients our bodies need to ingest in large supplies for us to survive. (The other two macros are carbohydrates and proteins.) Fat is critical for our bodies to function normally, and without it, we simply couldn't live. It's found not just underneath our skin (subcutaneous) and in our abdomens, but also in the cells in our brains and throughout the rest of our bodies, and around our vital organs (visceral fat). Some of this fat we are born with, but a lot of it we gather from the foods we eat. So let's take a look at the fat we're putting into our mouth.

Dietary Fat

- four major types of fats that are found in our food— saturated, monounsaturated, polyunsaturated, and trans
- chemical structures and physical properties are different, and tend to be divided between good fats and bad fats
- good fats are the monounsaturated and the polyunsaturated
- bad fats are the saturated and trans

The **unsaturated fats** are liquid at room temperature. They are predominantly found in foods from plants, such as vegetables, nuts, and seeds, as well as in fish. Think about the key ingredients you typically see in a Mediterranean diet. Unsaturated fats are considered good fats, because of their benefits, which include improving blood cholesterol levels (they lower the risk of heart disease and stroke), stabilizing heart rhythms, easing inflammation, and possibly lowering one's risk for developing rheumatoid arthritis. Unsaturated fats are further divided into two groups: monounsaturated and poly-unsaturated. The difference between the two is in their chemical structures. Without getting too scientific, both contain the same atoms—carbon, hydrogen, and oxygen—but how those atoms are arranged makes a difference. Monounsaturated fats contain only one double bond in its structure, while polyunsaturated fats contain two or more double bonds.

Good Sources of Monounsaturated Fats

- Cooking oils made from plants such as olive, peanut, soybean, sunflower, and canola
- Avocados
- Nuts such as almonds, hazelnuts, cashews, peanuts, and pecans
- Seeds such as pumpkin and sesame

Generally speaking, the more unsaturated a fat is, the better it is for your health. So, poly- (multiple) unsaturated fats are better than mono- (single) unsaturated, but both are drastically more benefi-cial than the saturated fats that we'll discuss shortly. Some oils, like canola, contain both monounsaturated and polyunsaturated fats. Most people don't consume enough healthful unsaturated fats. In fact, according to the American Heart Association, 8 to 10 percent of our daily calories should come from polyunsaturated fats. More evidence suggests that eating as much as 15 percent of daily calo-ries in the form of polyunsaturated fat in place of saturated fat can lower one's risk for heart disease.

Omega-3 fatty acids are the most "famous" of the polyunsatu-rated fats. They are considered "essential fats" because our bodies are unable to make them, so we must consume them in our food. Omega-3s have been shown to reduce inflammation, help with normal brain development and function, reduce symptoms of depression, improve heart health, decrease liver fat, prevent dementia, reduce asthma symptoms, and improve bone health, as well as reduce weight and waist size. Good sources of these fats are oily fish like salmon, mackerel, and herring, as well as oysters, sardines, flax seeds, chia seeds, walnuts, and soybeans. In fact, the World Health Organization (WHO) recommends eating at least two portions of oily fish per week to get sufficient amounts of the healthful omega-3 fats.

Good Sources of Polyunsaturated Fats

- Walnuts
- Sunflower seeds
- Soybeans
- Tofu
- Oils such as flax, corn, soybean, grapeseed, and safflower
- Fish such as salmon, mackerel, trout, sardines, herring, and albacore tuna

Saturated fats are quite different from unsaturated fats both in structure and impact on our health. From a chemical standpoint, these fats don't have any double bonds between their carbon molecules. This means they are *saturated* with hydrogen molecules, thus the term "saturated fats." Unlike unsaturated fats, saturated fats tend to be solid at room temperature.

The saturated fats have long been considered a "bad" fat, because they raise the LDL cholesterol (the bad type) in the body, which in turn can put one at a higher risk for heart disease and stroke. Recently, there has been conflicting data and messages about how bad saturated fats really are, but experts at the Harvard School of Public Health have deduced that cutting back on saturated fat can be good for health if people replace saturated fat with good fats, especially polyunsaturated fats. Evidence suggests that when someone eats good fats in place of the bad fats, they can lower the bad LDL cholesterol levels, which can ultimately lower the risk for heart disease.

While saturated fat is not the most healthful fat, it is still all right to have a small amount of it in your diet. The American Heart Association recommends that only 5 to 6 percent of your daily calories should come from saturated fat. What exactly does this mean? If you eat 2,000 calories in a day, no more than 120 calories should come from saturated fat. To put this number in terms of grams, that would be equivalent to 13 grams. Saturated fats are a natural component in many foods, the majority coming mainly from animal sources that include meat and dairy products.

Common Sources of Saturated Fats

- Fatty beef
- Poultry with skin
- Pork
- Lamb
- Cheese
- Tropical oil (coconut oil, palm oil, cocoa butter)
- Sour cream
- Butter
- Ice cream
- Lard and cream
- Other dairy products made from whole or 1 or 2% milk
- Cookies and other grain-based desserts

Trans fatty acids, commonly referred to as trans fats, got their comeuppance a long time ago when scientists and public health advocates rang the alarm about the potential and unnecessary dangers they can impose on our health.

Trans Fatty Acids

- Can be naturally occurring but are largely manufactured by companies.
- Are artificially synthesized via a process called hydrogenation: heating liquid vegetable oils in the presence of hydrogen gas and a catalyst (something that expedites the process). This process basically converts the oil into a solid, and thus you have a "partially hydrogenated" vegetable oil, which is more stable and less likely to spoil and become rancid.
- Margarine and shortening are the best examples of what trans fats look like in your kitchen.
- Partially hydrogenated oils became a favorite of the food industry because they're less likely to spoil and can withstand repeated heating without breaking down, thus making them ideal for frying fast foods.
- Trans fats flooded the market and could be found everywhere, including fried foods, processed snack foods, and baked goods.
- Dangers of trans fats:
  - They are the worst type of fat for the heart, blood vessels, and rest of the body.
  - They wreak internal havoc, including raising the bad LDL cholesterol and simultaneously lowering the good HDL cholesterol.
  - They increase inflammation.
  - They contribute to insulin resistance (make the insulin hormone less effective).
  - They damage the inner lining (endothelium) of blood vessels.

Not all trans fats are artificial. A relatively small amount occur naturally, and they are called ruminant trans fats, because they are found in meat and dairy that come from ruminant animals such as cattle, goats, and sheep. When ruminant animals eat grass, bacteria in their stomachs help digest the grass, and a byproduct of this process is the formation of trans fats. Natural trans fats come in modest amounts—2 to 6 percent of the fat in dairy products and 3 to 9 percent of the fat in certain cuts of lamb and beef. These trans fats that most of us consume from normal meat and dairy consumption should not be concerning, as studies have shown that moderate intake of these fats doesn't appear to be harmful. However, when it comes to the artificial trans fats, also known as partially hydrogenated oil or fat, consumer beware. These are hazardous to your health. International expert groups and public health authorities have recommended that we keep our trans fat consumption to less than 1 percent of our total energy intake. So, if you're consuming a 2,000-calorie diet, this is about 20 calories or 2 grams per day.

Look on the back of the food label and check to see if it contains trans fats. You should be aware that manufacturers use multiple terms to describe trans fats that can be confusing to the consumer. Make sure you look for these terms: trans fats, trans fatty acids, hydrogenated oil, and partially hydrogenated oils. If you see any of these terms, put the product back on the shelf and look for a similar product or different brand that doesn't contain any trans fats. There are plenty of companies that thankfully have altered their manufacturing processes and have significantly reduced or eliminated trans fats from their products. It's become such an important issue that many labels will clearly state right on the front of the package either *0g Trans Fats, No Trans Fats*, or *Trans Fat Free*.

Common Food Sources of Trans Fats

- Margarine
- Frozen pizza
- Baked goods such as cakes, cookies, crackers, and pies
- Fried foods such as French fries, donuts, and fried chicken
- Refrigerated dough such as biscuits and rolls
- Ready-to-use frostings
- Nondairy coffee creamer

Triglyceride Cheat Sheet

- Found in our food as well as made within our body.
- Chemical structure: comprised of three molecules of fatty acid joined with a molecule of glycerol (which is a type of alcohol).
- Comprise over 90 percent of all fats we consume; found in both animal and vegetable fats.
- Commonly found in butter, margarine, and oils such as vegetable, corn, and canola oil.
- Many types of triglycerides; some are saturated fats, while others are unsaturated fats.
- Our body also manufactures triglycerides. When we consume extra calories, alcohol, or sugar (carbohydrates), the liver takes these energy molecules and uses them to increase the production of triglycerides.
- When too many triglycerides float around in our blood, the excess is stored in our fat cells for later use when the body needs more energy.
- Most common type of fat in the body because of the frequent consumption, creation, and storage of triglycerides.

MACRONUTRIENTS AND THEIR CALORIES

Macronutrients are nutrients that the body needs in large amounts. These nutrients provide needed energy to the body in the form of calories. There are three macronutrients: fat, carbohydrate, and protein. We need all three of them for a healthy diet and proper nutrition.

- Fat: 9 calories per gram
- Carbohydrate: 4 calories per gram
- Protein: 4 calories per gram

Consuming and manufacturing some triglycerides is not a bad thing for our health. They are an extremely important source of energy. However, too many triglycerides in our blood can lead to serious health problems. They can cause the blood to become thicker and stickier, and this can lead to the blood forming too many clots, which can cause high blood pressure, heart disease, and stroke. High levels of triglycerides might also cause fatty liver disease and pancreatitis (inflammation of the pancreas).

Triglycerides and cholesterol are not the same thing, though some people tend to use the terms interchangeably. While both are fatty substances known by the general category name of lipids, chemically speaking, triglycerides are fats whereas cholesterol is not. Triglycerides are largely used by the body for energy purposes, while cholesterol plays a role in certain bodily functions such as hormone production and digestion. What is similar between the two is that both are found in the food we eat (like trans fats, cholesterol is also found in animal products) as well as being produced by the body. Cholesterol can't mix with or be dissolved in the blood, so the liver packages cholesterol with triglycerides and proteins in carrier molecules called lipoproteins.

The Fat Journey

Have you ever wondered how fat goes from your plate to your hips or abdomen or the back of your arms? Let's quickly take a trip to see how this happens. It all starts before you even put the fat in your mouth. When you look at that steak or donut, this releases chemicals like dopamine in your brain in anticipation of the satisfaction you are about to obtain. Your saliva glands go into overdrive and digestive enzymes are whipped into a frenzy, getting ready to start breaking down your fatty meal. The ultimate goal of your digestive system is to break the fat down into its most basic components: fatty acids and glycerol.

Once the fat hits your stomach, the enzyme lipase is thrown into the mix and helps to further break down the fat particles. The partially broken-down fat mix is sent to the small intestines, where more juices, enzymes, and other liquids like bile join the party and continue to emulsify (allow fat to mix with water) and continue the breakdown process. These tiny fat molecules are absorbed from the intestinal tract into the lymphatic system, which is a network of vessels similar to the circulatory system that carries blood throughout the body. Once the fat molecules are in the lymphatic system, they flow through the body until they eventually enter the bloodstream through large veins in the area of the chest. Now that these fatty molecules are in the blood system, they are free to go anywhere throughout the body.

The first important stop after entering the blood is the liver, the large organ located in the right-hand portion of the abdominal cavity, just beneath the diaphragm (breathing muscle) and on top of the stomach, right kidney, and intestines. The liver has many functions, including detoxification of the blood (cleaning it out) as well as assembling and manufacturing various molecules. The liver takes the pieces of fats and reassembles them into several products such as the good HDL cholesterol and triglycerides. Proteins are added to these fatty molecules so they can be carried to targeted destinations in the body, which include adipose (fat) cells and various organs like the brain, where they are incorporated into the cell membrane.

While too much body fat isn't good for us, we still need some fat, as it serves several important functions in the body, including: keeping us insulated and warm, storing important vitamins such as A, D, E, and K, storage of energy that can be used when the body needs it, and becoming an important structural component in the cell membranes that separate the inside of the cell from the outside.

An interesting fat fact is that we generally don't generate new fat cells after puberty. As we get heavier and accumulate more fat, the number of fat cells isn't growing, rather the size of the fat cells we already have simply gets bigger. (Two possible exceptions: there might be a production of more fat cells if an adult gains a significant amount of weight, or someone has liposuction performed where a large number of fat cells are removed, and the body responds by growing new ones.) The number of fat cells by the time we finish puberty will generally be a constant number that we will have for the rest of our lives. When you lose weight and "burn" fat, you are not reducing the number of fat cells; rather your body is shrinking the size of the fat cells. The process of gaining and losing weight typically means alternating between expanding and shrinking fat cells.

Body fat can be located in many places, but most commonly it's found underneath the skin (subcutaneous fat) and around the body's organs (visceral fat). Where your fat tends to accumulate has a lot to do with your gender and genetics. Women tend to carry it in their breasts, waist, hips, and buttocks. Men tend to see it

Types of Fat Tissue in the Body

WHITE FAT	BROWN FAT
• Most plentiful in the body. • Stores energy and vitamins. • Produces hormones like leptin that interact with the brain to get our body to eat less and burn more calories. (Leptin has the opposite effect of the hormone ghrelin, which is produced in the stomach and works with your brain to signal that you are hungry and need nourishment.) • Grows when we consume more calories than we burn, because when we eat food or drink beverages with calories, that intake of energy needs to go somewhere. It doesn't just disappear. • If the body doesn't have an immediate demand to use energy—such as energy needed to complete a two-mile walk or climb the stairs to get to the bedroom—then it needs to go somewhere. That somewhere is into your fat cells. • When the body has unused fat, glucose, and protein circulating in the blood, the insulin hormone will act on the fat cell and cause it to take them up and convert them to fat molecules and store them as fat droplets. This is how the fat cells get bigger. The more fatty acids, protein, and glucose circulating around, the more ingredients that will enter the cell to be converted into fat.	• Often called the "good" fat. • Much less abundant in the body than white fat. • Mostly found in newborn babies, between the shoulders. • As we grow and mature, the percentage of brown fat greatly diminishes until it's almost nonexistent. • The main function of this fat is something called thermogenesis—the production of heat. • Newborn babies produce heat by breaking down fat molecules into the smaller fatty acids. Once a newborn starts eating more, the calories that go unused get stored in the developing layer of white fat cells, and eventually, the brown fat starts to go away and the white cells grow, which is why adults have very little or no brown fat at all.

accumulate in the chest, abdomen, and buttocks. Our genes, which we can't change, intricately program where this excess fat likes to set up shop and call home.

Burn the Fat

There is one underlying principle when it comes to fat burning or shrinkage that has not changed and remains fundamental. Reducing the amount of body fat occurs when the energy demands from the body exceed the amount of energy that is readily available. Think about your car running out of gas. Your car will not be able to run without gas—its energy source. So what do you do? You go to the gas station, purchase fuel, fill up your tank, and drive away to go on about your business. The body encounters a similar situation when it is low on fuel, except rather than go to a gas station, the body reaches into its stores of fat, which are large reserves of energy that can be accessed and used when needed.

To transition into the fat-burning mode, the body does two things. First, the body stops storing excess or unused energy into the fat stores. Second, the body uses the energy *already* stored in the fat cells to meet its energy demand. Our brain senses that our energy demands are not being met or close to not being met and triggers a series of chemical messages that finally arrive to the fat cell, instructing it to release fatty acid molecules into the bloodstream. Various organs throughout the body pick up these fatty acid molecules, break them apart, then use the energy that was stored in these chemical bonds to carry out the activities they need to perform. This repeated release of energy from the fat cell eventually causes it to shrink, and when enough shrinkage occurs it can be seen in one's appearance as well as the decreasing numbers on the scale.

There are two equations that lie at the center of weight loss and fat burning:

Weight Loss Equation
ENERGY IN (Food) < ENERGY OUT (Calories burned)
Fat Burning Equation
ENERGY AVAILABLE < ENERGY NEEDED

In the **FAST BURN** plan, we are going to work on both equations, which will help you both lose weight and burn fat. The key to altering the equations is energy demand. You must increase your energy demand to make sure that the energy you're taking in is less than the energy you're burning off. Increasing energy demand will also drive the body to refuel by depleting its fat stores and thus shrinking the amount of body fat. Over the next nine weeks, we are going to attack the issue in four ways that will accelerate the burn.

FAST BURN Strategies

1. **Time-restricted feeding method of intermittent fasting.** This will help lower the energy available and increase the energy demand, sending the body searching for the energy stored in our fat.

2. **Exercise and other physical activity.** We are not going to be going to the gym for hours and hours on end. That can be one effective strategy for some, but the average person likely doesn't have the ability, time, desire, or environmental conditions to do this. We are, however, going to increase activity in a doable way that will definitely in-

crease our energy demand (energy needed), an important part of the fat burning equation.

3. **Calorie reduction and improved calorie quality.** This doesn't mean that you are going to be hungry or that you will only be eating fruits and vegetables. It does, however, mean that you will be eating cleaner foods that are still tasty and fun, but better for your health and not packed with unnecessary calories and processed ingredients. There will be flexibility in the food choices presented to you so that a broad range of dietary preferences and restrictions that you might have can be accommodated.

4. **Clean eating.** Not only will you do intermittent fasting, but you will also add an element of clean eating, where many of the foods you eat will have less processed ingredients and thus less chance of disrupting hormones, increasing blood sugars, and exhausting some of your body's important organs. Eating cleaner (not perfect) as you fast is a way to maximize the benefits as well as expedite your weight loss.

In order for our bodies to function properly, we need a certain amount of fat in foods and a certain amount to be stored in our bodies. The goal of **FAST BURN** is not to eliminate all fats, but to increase the consumption of good fats, decrease the consumption of bad fats, and reduce the amount and location of body fat so that we feel better, look better, and prevent the onset or delay the progression of disease. If you follow the plan with these principles in mind, you can surely achieve results that make you proud.

2

The Power of
Intermittent Fasting

INTERMITTENT FASTING (IF) HAS BEEN ONE OF THE WORLD'S hottest trends in weight loss management and fat reduction, and for good reason. There has been anecdotal evidence from millions of people that it can be extremely effective, and convincing research has confirmed that IF can make a difference not only on the scale but also in other important biometrics, such as blood pressure, cholesterol levels, and insulin resistance.

Intermittent fasting is when you alternate between periods of fasting and periods of eating. In most variations of this plan, you are typically not told what to eat, but rather when you can and cannot eat. When you think about the history of our consumption patterns, in many ways early man regularly followed intermittent fasting. Food was not available in large quantities year-round for many, and today's modern conveniences of grocery stores and refrigerators to keep things from spoiling during warm weather were nonexistent. When the hunter-gatherers couldn't find anything to eat on their forage, they went without food if they didn't have anything stored. This ability to go for sometimes long periods of time without food and still function well was an evolutionary adaptation our ancestors made that benefits us today. It's important to be clear that IF doesn't mean you are going to be starving or going for days on end without eating. That is not the intention of IF, nor is it a safe nutritional strategy. Food is not a luxury for the body; it is an absolute necessity. We get our energy and nutrients that we need to survive from our food. Unfortunately, we often consume too much food, and this has led to the skyrocketing rates of obesity and its numerous health-related consequences.

IF is a way to introduce more order and discipline into our eating patterns. It gives us the opportunity to appreciate food and not take it for granted like we often do when we can reach and grab whatever is closest whenever we get the urge, even if we're not hungry. Some studies have shown that people who follow an IF style of eating tend to be less hungry overall and do a better job of distributing their calorie consumption over the hours that comprise their eating or feeding window.

As with most popular trends, there are lots of derivative methods when it comes to IF. People are taking the basic tenets of the concept and making modifications—some good, some not so good— and still calling it IF. When it comes to health and your safety, it's important to consider those methods or strategies that have decent science and strong anecdotal evidence behind them. Let's review some of these methods so that you can put them to best use over the next nine weeks.

Time-Restricted Feeding (TRF)

This is one of the most popular IF methods and is quite simple to understand. You restrict the times each day that you eat and the times you are not going to eat (fast). You basically form a feeding or eating window and a fasting window. Together, these windows need to add up to 24 hours. For example, you might decide to do a 12-hour feeding window. Well, that means you are also planning to do a 12-hour fast. Now that you have decided you're going to do a 12:12 program, you then decide the times you want the fasting and feeding windows to start and stop. Let's say you wake up at 7 A.M., and you typically eat breakfast at 8 A.M. This would mean your feeding window starts at 8 A.M. To give yourself a 12-hour feeding window, this means you would stop eating at 8 P.M. Your fasting window would be just the opposite. You would start fasting at 8 P.M. and not eat anything until 8 A.M. the next morning.

Millions of people have tried this method. Many report that the first few days take some adjustments, particularly being able to stick to the feeding and fasting windows and making sure you resist the urge to prematurely break the fast by eating when you're not supposed to. Therefore, it's best to start with something like the 12:12 schedule, then over the course of several weeks work your way up to the more aggressive fasting schedules if that's what you desire and are capable of. While you might be excited about trying an aggressive schedule, remember that you need to give your body time to adjust to this new style of eating, so be patient. The most obvious way to experience the least amount of life disruption and inconvenience with this type of fast is to make sure you are sleeping during some or most of the fasting window. If you sleep eight hours and it's during your fast, then it means you really only have an active fast of four hours, which you will probably find is not at all difficult to follow.

There are all kinds of variations on the guidelines when it comes to TRF, but one that I have found very useful is the allowance of 50 calories or less during your fasting window. It's best to have these calories in the form of liquid beverages such as flavored water, tea, or coffee, but it's important not to exceed 50 calories total during the entire fasting period. Keeping it at 50 or less means you won't break the fast, but exceeding this limit means there's a good chance you will break it and your body will switch away from the fat-burning and use the food/beverage calories instead, because they are much easier and more convenient to use. If you want to be a "purist" when it comes to the fast, then don't consume any calories at all during your fasting window. I don't believe the 50 calories will have much of an effect in limiting your results, but some people like to be hard-core, and if that's your profile, by all means feel free to take that path.

Research suggests that the longer or more aggressive your fasting window, the more likely you are to experience some of the benefits, especially weight loss and fat reduction. There are some who will do a 16:8 or an 18:6. In all transparency, these schedules are not the easiest to follow and definitely not for beginners, but anecdotal evidence as well as extrapolating from the principles of IF suggest that this degree of fasting would possibly produce more dramatic results in a shorter timeframe. It's important, however, that you choose fasting and feeding windows that you know you will be able to maintain and not feel like you're going too long without nutrition and seriously struggling to hang on. If you find yourself getting weak or lightheaded or dizzy, then it's possible that either the fast window you've chosen is too long, or you are not eating enough during your feeding window to help carry you through the fast. Make the necessary adjustments so that you are not endangering yourself. If it means you need to have a shorter window, that's completely fine. Our bodies are not the same, so we respond differently; no one knows your body better than you do.

Fasting/Feeding Options

TRF 12:12		
FASTING	➡	FEEDING
8 P.M. —8 A.M.		8 P.M. —8 A.M.

TRF 14:10		
FASTING	➡	FEEDING
8 P.M. —10 A.M.		10 A.M.—8 P.M.

TRF 16:8		
FASTING	➡	FEEDING
8 P.M. —12 P.M.		12 P.M. —8 P.M.

TRF 18:6		
FASTING	➡	FEEDING
8 P.M. —2 P.M.		2 P.M.—8 P.M.

5:2 Method

Another popular IF method is the 5:2, where you eat how you would normally eat for five days, and for two days you fast. There are two versions of this method, the difference being in how you conduct your fasting days. In the first version, during the two fasting days you keep your total calorie count to a maximum of 500 calories per day. Some make it a little less restrictive and give you latitude to go up to 800 calories. The five other days you don't count calories and eat what you want with a focus on eating more healthful foods. It's advised that the two fasting days not be consecutive, so you should have at least one non-fasting day in between. In the second version of this method, you eat normally for the five days, but the two fasting days are days of no calories at all. This method is a lot more difficult, since you are fasting for twenty-four hours two times a week. See the sample 5:2 schedule below.

Alternate Day

This IF method rolls out exactly as its name implies—every other day you do a fast. There are some variations, however, when it

5:2 Intermittent Fasting

MONDAY	TUESDAY	WEDNESDAY	THURSDAY	FRIDAY	SATURDAY	SUNDAY
Normal	Normal	Fast	Normal	Normal	Fast	Normal

Alternate Day Intermittent Fasting

MONDAY	TUESDAY	WEDNESDAY	THURSDAY	FRIDAY	SATURDAY	SUNDAY
Normal	Total Fast or 500 cals	Normal	Total Fast or 500 cals	Normal	Total Fast or 500 cals	Normal

comes to the fasting day. Some will avoid all solid foods for the full twenty-four hours, while others will allow up to a total of 500 or so calories. During the feeding days, there are no caloric restrictions and people tend to eat whatever and how much they want. One small study that looked at this method found that the participants lost an average of eleven pounds over a twelve-week period, which is not fast weight loss, but respectable.

While the alternate method appears to have some promise, it's criticized in some circles because it's relatively extreme and the likelihood of most people being able to follow it for a sustained period of time is quite low compared to the other IF options. Also, if you have underlying medical conditions, think twice before trying this, as those fasting days can be quite stressful to the body given the lack of nutrient intake. This fasting method would not be suggested for someone who is just beginning their IF journey. A sample schedule for this alternate method appears above.

24-Hour Fast

This method involves a full day of fasting from solid foods. People are allowed, however, to drink water, tea, and other calorie-free drinks during their fasting period. Some people will do just one twenty-four-hour fast a week, whereas others who are more ambitious will do two. On the non-fasting days, people are expected to resume normal eating, but still be mindful of not consuming too many calories. This method is not for the faint of heart. There have been complaints of headaches, fatigue, and increased irritability in the early phases of following this plan. The reports, however, go on to say that these early complaints diminish as users adjusted and their bodies acclimated to the schedule. A sample schedule of this method is shown below.

Regardless of which method you choose, one thing is certain: to maximize results, it's extremely helpful to eat healthful foods that are cleaner and not full of processed ingredients. It's a mistake to think that consuming as many calories as you want during your feeding windows or days is not going to diminish your results. Some people erroneously think that the fasting period/day is almost magical and allows them to eat whatever they want and still see great

24 hour fast

MONDAY	TUESDAY	WEDNESDAY	THURSDAY	FRIDAY	SATURDAY	SUNDAY
Normal	Normal	24-HR FAST	Normal	Normal	24-HR FAST	Normal

results at the end of the week. Not true. The old-fashioned rule that calories in must be less than calories out still applies. The quality of the food you eat also matters. Processed foods, beyond tending to have more calories in them, can be disruptive to our hormonal system as well as our digestive process, and these conditions can prevent effective weight loss.

Benefits of Intermittent Fasting

Like many popular dieting or nutritional trends, sometimes it can be very difficult to separate fact from fiction, real science from pseudoscience. The good news about intermittent fasting, however, is that the science and researchers appear to be catching up to the demand for information and some of the claims that users have made. Current research has suggested that some of the benefits of IF include weight loss, improved brain health, reduced inflammation, reduced risk of chronic conditions, improved health markers, and reduced asthma symptoms. Let's take a closer look at some of these benefits.

Potential Benefits of Intermittent Fasting

- Weight loss
- Decreased belly fat
- Decreased inflammation
- Improved asthma-related symptoms
- Improved brain health
- Preserved learning and memory functioning
- Improved health markers
- Reduced insulin resistance

- Reduced risk of chronic conditions
- Autophagy
- Telomere lengthening (protecting chromosomes and lengthening life)

Weight Loss

Of course, weight loss is at the top of most people's list of reasons to do IF. Anecdotal reports of weight loss success are widespread and vigorous at all levels of IF. One of the ways IF might drive weight loss is by lowering the body's levels of the insulin hormone. When we eat food, the body breaks down the carbohydrates into glucose, which then can be used by our cells for energy. If the energy isn't used right away, the glucose is brought to the fat cells and gets stored as fat so that it can be broken down later when energy is needed. The insulin hormone is what allows the cells to uptake the glucose. When we eat food, the insulin levels rise, because something needs to be done with all of the glucose that is about to start circulating in our blood. When we are not eating, the insulin levels drop, because its actions are no longer in great demand.

The reasoning then goes something like this: when we are fasting—that is, not consuming calories—then we are no longer breaking down carbohydrates and releasing glucose into the blood. If there's no glucose, there's no need for insulin. But our body still needs energy to live and function, even if we aren't eating or haven't eaten recently. So where will it get the energy from? Well, the body has a limited number of places where it stores glucose—the liver and muscles—and it stores the glucose in a form called glycogen. So, when the body needs energy and there is no energy available in the food, the body calls on the liver and muscles to break down the glycogen and release that glucose. This is a good solution for energy demand, but unfortunately, this glycogen storage is limited, and the body will exhaust its supply. So what next? That's where the fat takes center stage.

The body's chemical messengering system detects that it is low on fuel and there is little or no storage left in the tank. It needs emergency fuel. The body remembers that it stored excess glucose in the fat cells, so it calls on the fat to break down and release the glucose. Once this happens, the body now has energy it can use. The body will keep breaking down that fat as long as you need energy and you have no other source from which you can get it. However, when you start eating food again, the body will stop breaking down the fat and instead use the food for energy. It's much easier for the body to use food for energy than it is to break down the fat, which is a complicated, time-consuming, inefficient, and multistep process. So, it stands to reason that the longer you stay in the fasting state, the longer your body will need to break down fat to meet its energy needs. This is supported by reports that people who have longer fast windows, up to 16 and 18 hours, experience more dramatic weight loss and greater body fat percentage dropped. The underlying weight loss principle of IF is to get our insulin levels low enough and hold them there long enough that our bodies have no choice but to burn fat.

Improve Brain Function

Early research suggests that going without food for a period of time increases your brain's natural growth factors such as brain-derived neurotrophic factor (BDNF), and these in turn support the survival and growth of the brain cells called neurons. There's something called "metabolic switching," which means the body's fuel source alternates between glucose and ketones (chemicals made by the liver when it burns fat). There are reports that when the body is switching between these energy sources, our mental capabilities are the sharpest and degenerative diseases are slowed. One study found that metabolic switching can promote resistance of the brain to injury and disease.

While glucose is the brain's primary and preferred fuel, when it's not available, the liver breaks down fats into several products, including ketones. When these ketones are available, they are the utilized energy source. Higher ketone levels have been linked to improved learning, memory, and cognition. It's thought by some that ketones might actually provide more energy to neurons than glucose, and this boost in effective energy allows the brain cells to more adequately slow the process of cellular death and brain deterioration.

Researchers have examined this principle in animal studies and found slower cognitive decline and increased brain cell longevity. Because of these promising studies in animals, there are serious implications when it comes to IF potentially preventing or slowing down the progression of Alzheimer's disease. Scientists are now conducting this research in humans to see if what they have found in animals will also be confirmed in humans.

While ketones can be used by the body for energy, a word of caution is imperative. Too many ketones in the body can be extremely harmful. High levels of ketones can lead to dehydration and cause a chemical change in the blood, causing it to become acidic. This state is called ketoacidosis and it can lead to coma and, when completely out of control, even death. This can be particularly threatening in the case of diabetics who have poor sugar control and utilization. Because their insulin hormone is either ineffective or they don't make enough of it, they are unable to take up the glucose into the cells, and thus can't take advantage of it as energy. So, they break down fats instead and use the ketones for energy.

Reduced Inflammation

Inflammation is an extremely important process in the body as it responds to potential infection and disease. When the body encounters foreign substances, our white blood cells, which are part of our immune system, release disease-fighting chemicals into the blood and affected tissues. This chemical release leads to increased blood flow to the area that's infected or injured, which is why you might see redness or feel warmth. This increased blood flow delivers more immune fighters to the area as the body launches a defense and attacks the foreign invader. In order for us to stay healthy, we need a strong immune system and we need to be able to quickly respond to injury or foreign invaders. However, there can be too much of a good thing. Inflammation that is out of control or inappropriate can cause damage to otherwise healthy tissue.

When you have chronic and sustained inflammation, this all-important inflammatory response can cause serious damage to healthy cells, tissues, and organs. When cells are repeatedly and severely harmed, the DNA can be damaged, tissues can be destroyed, and internal scarring can occur. Excessive inflammation has been linked to several diseases, including heart disease, rheumatoid arthritis, type 2 diabetes, obesity, asthma, neurodegenerative diseases, and cancer.

Certain drugs have been helpful at reducing inflammation, including nonsteroidal anti-inflammatory drugs (NSAIDs) like aspirin, ibuprofen, and naproxen. Steroids are also effective at suppressing the immune system, along with certain supplements that contain fish oil, lipoic acid, and curcumin. But researchers now believe that IF can be another way to reduce this harmful inflammation. It's believed to do this by reducing monocytes, the cells in the blood that cause inflammation. It appears that the monocytes were less inflammatory in people who were fasting compared to those who weren't.

Chronic Conditions Risk Reduction

When researchers look at the impact that treatment or other interventions have on one's risk of developing disease, they often look at certain markers that are predictive of what conditions might develop or resolve. Some risk markers that IF has been shown to lower include high cholesterol levels, reduced insulin resistance, and decreased blood pressure. These markers are associated with a variety of chronic conditions, including diabetes, heart disease, and stroke.

Autophagy

This scientific principle simply means self-eating (*auto*: self; *phage*: eat). In the absence of external food sources, the body eats itself by destroying and then recycling its own damaged cell bits and proteins, to make way for newer and healthier versions to be built. Scientists believe that autophagy is essential in helping protect against several diseases, including cancer, dementia, and Parkinson's disease.

In the **FAST BURN** plan, IF is an important element. It will help deliver all the benefits previously mentioned and help you not only reach your goals faster, but also maintain your success. We will be using the TRF *and* 5:2 methods over the next nine weeks. If you're a beginner, I suggest you start with the 12:12 method. Try this for a couple of weeks, and if you feel like you can be a little more aggressive with your fasting window and really stick to it, then I encourage you to move to the 14:10 method to finish out the first part of the plan. For the second part of the plan, consider going to the 16:8 for as much of the last four weeks as you can. If you have already tried IF and you are accustomed to a more aggressive fasting window such as 14 or 16 hours, feel free to start with that instead of the 12. You can always choose a more aggressive option when it comes to the schedule if you are able to handle it.

There are a few things I want you to keep in mind as you go

through the plan. First, once you choose your fasting and feeding windows, you really need to stick to them for at least a week. Don't change up day to day or every couple of days. By that I mean, don't do 12:12 on Monday, then go to 14:10 for the next couple of days, then go back to 12:12 the following day. Your body needs time to adjust to the schedule, so shifting it frequently will not give it the time it needs to make the necessary adjustments and help deliver the results you want.

If you find that you have chosen a fasting/feeding schedule that is too difficult to follow, you can downgrade your schedule. Let's say you chose a 14:10 and you find it too difficult. Simply go down to 12:12. What's most important in all of this is that you stick to your windows and not break them. This is not about bragging rights or projecting a certain image to your friends. There's no value or honor in choosing a challenging schedule just to be able to tell others that you are going hard-core, when in reality you are not following the plan because it's too difficult. It's much better to focus on choosing what works for you, something that will challenge you but be achievable at the same time.

Remember that during a fast, water is your friend. Expanding your stomach with no calories is the best way to make it through the fast should you have a sudden urge to eat or you crave a particular food. You are still allowed 50 calories maximum during your fasting window, so feel free to get those from flavored water, tea, and/or coffee, but make sure you are keeping track so you don't exceed the 50-calorie ceiling. Also, make use of sugarless gum. Chewing gum can help you outlast a craving and help prevent you from eating when you're supposed to be fasting.

Now that you understand fat and how it can shrink, and now that you understand the workings and benefits of IF, it's time to get your body to **FAST BURN!** I have tried to lay out the meal plan simply to be sure it's straightforward and clear. Do the best you can to follow the plan and the instructions as closely as possible. I have designed **FAST BURN** to be a "forgiving program," which means that if you make a mistake or mess up a little in what you eat or when you eat, it is not going to penalize you, and you don't need to start all over again. Just take a deep breath, refocus, and go on to the next meal or next time period.

The signature smoothie of this plan is **The Burner Smoothie** (page 254), crafted with specific ingredients to fill you up on fewer calories while increasing your metabolism to facilitate fat burning. It takes only minutes to make this drink, and it's not only full of powerful nutrients, but also delicious and portable. You can make it and store it in the fridge or freezer and take it with you. This drink is so powerful and effective that you can have it anytime you want in place of a meal. Your body will be grateful for all of the tremendous energy it provides and how well it keeps hunger at bay.

This plan has three parts that are followed in order. Each part has its own underlying principles as to how it helps you burn fat. Each week in each part has its own set of guidelines, so you need to pay attention to those guidelines for that particular week. These guidelines are not random or haphazard. I have designed them the way they are written for particular reasons, some of which you might or might not understand. To find success, you must believe in the plan, believe in the process, and, most important, believe in yourself. If you want to read through the entire plan or read ahead a couple of weeks to see what's to come, by all means do so. It can help you organize better and prepare yourself mentally when you know what to expect and when to expect it.

Part I—Ignition

IGNITION is the first four weeks of the plan. It is designed to acclimate you to a new style and schedule of eating. The pace of the entire program is fast, so be prepared to hit the ground running. The better and quicker you adhere to the guidelines of the program, the faster you will see results. It's important to note that the entire program has been constructed in a way to allow the greatest flexibility and yet still deliver results. There will be times when you will have the opportunity to choose the item or items you select for a meal or snack. If none of the choices fit your eating style (if you're a vegan or vegetarian or pescatarian) or you have a medical condition you need to be sensitive to (for example, you need to eat gluten-free), then make the necessary substitutions, but please do so wisely. If you want fish instead of grilled chicken, the correct substitution is not fried catfish; rather, it's grilled or baked fish. If all the substitutions are not clearly spelled out for you, simply remember the spirt of the program, which is to eat cleaner, less-processed ingredients and reduce unnecessary calories that come in fried foods, cream sauces, and sugary foods.

Part II—Intermission

Intermission is the halfway point of the program. It's one week that is specially designed to give your body and mind a rest. It's meant to give you a chance to reset and take a breather. This week is all about maintenance. You've built up momentum to this point, and so we want to keep it going by allowing you time to assess your progress and make the mental adjustments to attack the last part of the program.

Part III—Acceleration

During **ACCELERATION**, as its name implies, you are going to really put your foot on the gas for the next four weeks. They will be challenging, but they won't be difficult to the point where you're frustrated and feel like you can't follow the plan. If you want great results, then you must give great effort. Remember the basic tenet of any plan, "You get out of it what you put into it." These last four weeks are all about giving it your all and putting forth your best effort. You started this plan with goals and expectations, and these four weeks combined with your previous work can help you achieve these goals. The principles underlying **ACCELERATION** are additive to those for **IGNITION**. The plan builds on what you've already been doing and gives you new strategies to continue your weight loss and transformation. Work hard and the results will come.

PART I

Ignition

3

Week 1:

Transition

WEIGH YOURSELF IN THE MORNING BEFORE STARTING the week and record it. Don't weigh yourself throughout the week; rather, weigh only once a week, so your next weigh-in will be the same day the following week in the morning. Weigh yourself in the same manner as you did in the beginning. Wear the same clothes or type of clothes each time you weigh in, or if you prefer to wear no clothes at all while weighing in, you can do that. The key is that you must be consistent in your weighing procedure. It's also important to use the same scale for every weigh-in, as scales can differ by as much as several pounds, which means your results will be inaccurate and not reflective of your hard work.

This week you are going to follow the 12:12 IF method. You choose the starting and ending times for your 12-hour fasting window and 12-hour feeding window. (Refer back to chapter 2 to be reminded of how to do this.) During your fasting window, try not to go long stretches without eating, as it is better to keep your calories as evenly distributed as possible to prevent overconsumption of calories and insulin spikes. Try to eat something—whether it's a meal or snack—about every three hours to avoid getting too hungry and making poor decisions. It's important that even though you're in your feeding window, you eat slowly and mindfully enough that you can not only taste and enjoy your meals and snacks, but notice your body's cues that you are full. Don't eat until you're so full that you "can't eat another bite." If you need less than what's recommended for a particular meal or snack, then great, go ahead and eat less, which is even better.

Based on your location and access to certain foods, you might find yourself unable to get the foods that are listed as meal 2 options, but you have access to foods listed for meal 3. Feel free to go ahead and make the switch and eat meal 3 in the time slot for meal 2 and vice versa. Note that while this switching is permitted, try not to do it more than a few times a week if you can help it. A strategy that will help keep you on track is preparation. Take a few minutes either the day before or at the start of the week and formulate a game plan for what your meal choices will be and the foods you'll need to make them. If you know you have a meeting on your schedule, or you know you'll be in a situation that will make accessing the foods you need difficult, form a contingency plan early so that you're not stuck and unable to get what you need to stick to the plan. The same can be said for the daily exercise suggestion. If you are aware that there is a day or two during which it will be difficult to complete the exercise, feel free to move the exercises around to fit your schedule. For example, if there's exercise scheduled for day 2 and you know you'll be traveling all day and simply won't have the necessary time to do and complete the exercise, go ahead and swap that day's exercise activities with a rest day.

Feel free to make some slight adjustments in the meal schedule that you find in the daily meal plans. Maybe you can't fit in all of the meals or simply are hungry enough to eat all of the food listed. That is completely fine. If you're not hungry, by all means don't force yourself to eat. However, do your best to distribute your meals as evenly as possible throughout your feeding window. You don't want to skip a meal and then double up on the next one. This can cause non-beneficial spikes in your hormones like insulin, and one of the important things you want to be mindful of is keeping your hormone levels as even as possible.

Throughout the plan, you'll often see a direction for you to have a "serving" of fruit. A serving of fruit generally means a piece of fruit about the size of your fist—an apple, peach, nectarine, or orange, ½ cup berries, a small (6-inch) banana, sixteen grapes, half a grapefruit, or ¼ cup dried fruit or ¼ cup 100 percent fresh fruit juice. Note that dried fruit is allowed as long as it's 100 percent natural with no added sugar and as long as you're eating the equivalent in dried fruit to a piece of fresh fruit the size of your fist. You will also see suggestions for snacks in the daily meal plans, but if you don't like what is listed or don't have it, simply turn to chapter 14 and choose a snack based on the calorie guidelines that are listed.

Throughout the plan, you'll be given the option of a smoothie or protein shake. For the purposes of this book, the two are interchangeable. The key is to follow the recommended calorie count regardless of which one you choose. Making this substitution increases the flexibility of the plan.

Guidelines

- You can have 1 glass of wine or 1 lite beer four out of the seven days. You can't, however, save them up and drink all four in one day or even two in one day. It's one per day for four days.
- If you don't eat meat, make substitutions appropriately with fish or vegetables.
- Soups can be consumed with 2 saltine crackers if desired.
- Burritos can be homemade or frozen. If you opt for a frozen burrito, make sure it's a low-sodium variety (300 mg or less per serving).
- If a sandwich calls for cheese, it should be 1 slice of cheese of your choice and the size should be approximately 3½ inches square, which is the typical size of packaged cheese.

- You are allowed 50 calories maximum during your fasting window, so feel free to get those from flavored water, herbal tea, and/or coffee, but make sure you are keeping track so you don't exceed the 50-calorie capacity for the entire window.

- You must consume 1 cup water before eating a meal; you must consume 1 cup water during your meal. You can add lemon or lime to your water, and you can drink fizzy water if you desire. This water is meant only to be flavored by fresh fruit, not pre-flavored by the manufacturer. Pre-flavored drinks often contain chemicals and other processed ingredients that can interfere with your hormones and weight loss efforts.

- You can drink coffee, but only 1 small cup per day. Stay away from all those fancy coffee preparations that have lots of calories. Your coffee should contain no more than 50 calories.

- Don't eat your first meal until two hours after you wake up.

- Do not eat the last meal within two hours of going to sleep. You can eat a 100-calorie snack before going to bed if desired.

- Be smart when you choose snacks. Avoid chips and donuts and candy; you can have them some of the time, but don't eat them often. If you must have something like these items, make it only one of your snacks for the day and find healthier options for the other snacks.

- You don't have to eat all the food on the day's menu if you don't want to, but no skipping meals, no doubling up on meals, and no exceeding the meal guidelines in size and volume.

- Condiments such as ketchup, mayo, and mustard are

allowed, but no more than 2 tablespoons at each meal for ketchup and mustard and 1 tablespoon for mayo; 2 to 3 tablespoons low-sodium soy sauce is allowed.

- Spices are unlimited.
- While fresh fruit is always preferred, canned and frozen fruit are allowed. Just make sure they are water-based and there are no added sugars.
- Canned and frozen vegetables are allowed. Please be aware of the sodium content. Try for low sodium: 140 mg or less per serving.
- You are allowed as much plain or fizzy water as you like per day.
- Flavored waters are allowed, but keep them at 60 calories or less per day.
- 1 bottle of sports drink is allowed per day, but keep it at 60 calories or less.
- 1 cup freshly squeezed lemonade per day.
- 1 cup juice (not from concentrate) per day.
- 1 cup unsweetened iced tea or herbal tea per day.
- 1 cup 1% or 2% milk, unsweetened soy milk, or unsweetened almond milk per day.
- 1 cup coffee with minimal sugar (½ teaspoon), milk (2 tablespoons), or half-and-half (1 tablespoon).
- NO white bread (100% whole-grain or 100% whole-wheat bread allowed).
- NO soda (diet or regular).
- NO fried food.
- NO white pasta (except in the case of chicken noodle soup).
- Five of the seven days you must do some type of cardiovascular exercise, commonly called cardio.

Pay attention to the guidelines written for that day. If you need to exercise on different days than listed, then go ahead and do that as long as you get five days of cardio-related physical activity in a seven-day period.

| | | | | | | | | | | | | | | | **DAY 1** | | | | | | | | | | | | | | | | |

Meal 1

- 1 cup lemon water: Pour 8 ounces water, either hot or cold. Squeeze the juice from half a lemon directly into the water.
- 1 piece of fruit. This can be 1 banana, 1 apple, 1 pear, etc. It can also be ½ cup raspberries, blueberries, blackberries, or strawberries.

Choose one of the following:
- small bowl of oatmeal (1½ cups cooked)
- 2 egg whites or 1 egg-white omelet with diced veggies (made with 2 egg whites max)
- 1 small bowl of sugar-free cereal with fat-free, skim, or 1% or 2% milk
- ½ cup fresh juice *not* from concentrate (grapefruit, apple, orange juice, tomato, carrot, etc.)

Snack 1

- Any fast snack

Meal 2

- Large green garden salad with only 2 tablespoons fat-free dressing, no bacon bits, no croutons. Keep it clean. You can add 3 ounces chicken or fish if desired.

Snack 2

- Any item 100 calories or less

Meal 3

Choose one of the following:
- 6-ounce piece of grilled or baked chicken or fish with 2 servings of veggies

- 4 servings of vegetables with ½ cup brown rice
- Tender Baked Pork Chops (see recipe, page 273), with 2 servings of veggies

Snack 3

- Any item 100 calories or less

Exercise

30 minutes of cardiovascular activity. You can do it all in one session or you can break it up into two different sessions. Choose a combination of the items below to fulfill your exercise requirement.

Gym Options

- 15 minutes of walking/running on treadmill
- 15 minutes on elliptical machine
- 15 minutes on stationary bicycle
- 15 minutes of swimming laps
- 15 minutes on stair climber
- 15 minutes of spinning
- 15 minutes of rowing machine
- 15 minutes of treadmill intervals

Non-gym Options

- 15 minutes of jogging outside
- 225 jump rope revolutions
- 15 minutes of brisk walking
- 15 minutes of walking up and down a staircase of at least 10 stairs. Walking up and down the staircase is considered 1 set (rest between sets as needed).
- 15 minutes of Zumba
- 15 minutes of riding bicycle outside

- 15 minutes of hiking
- 15 minutes of any other high-intensity cardio
- 15 minutes of alternating between running and walking. Run for 1 minute, then walk for 1 minute, then run again and walk again. Repeat the cycle for 15 minutes.

| | | | | | | | | | | | | | | | **DAY 2** | | | | | | | | | | | | | | | | | |

Meal 1

- 1 cup lemon water: Pour 8 ounces water, either hot or cold. Squeeze the juice from half a lemon directly into the water.

Choose one of the following (must be 300 calories or less):
- 1 fruit smoothie such as Tropical Dash Smoothie (see recipe, page 285)
- 1 veggie smoothie (any veggies you want)
- 1 protein shake

Snack 1

Choose one of the following:
- 14 raw almonds
- ½ cucumber, sliced, with 2 tablespoons hummus
- 8 baby carrots with 2 tablespoons hummus
- 1 celery stalk, cut into slices, with 2 tablespoons hummus

Meal 2

Choose one of the following:
- 3 servings of vegetables. Remember, a serving is about the size of the average person's fist. One of the vegetables must be a dark-green leafy vegetable, such as spinach, kale, lettuce, mustard greens, collard greens, chicory, or Swiss chard.
- Large green salad (all or any of the following: lettuce 5 olives, 3 tablespoons shredded cheese, 5 cherry tomatoes, 2 tablespoons nuts, sliced cucumbers) with 2 tablespoons low-fat or fat-free vinaigrette-type dressing and 3 ounces sliced chicken or ½ cup beans if desired; no bacon bits and no croutons)
- 1 cup brown rice or quinoa with ¾ cup beans

Snack 2

- Any item 150 calories or less

Meal 3

Choose one of the following. Your choice must be different from your selection for meal 2.

- Large green garden salad (no croutons, no bacon bits) with 2 tablespoons fat-free or low-fat vinaigrette dressing and optional 3 ounces diced or sliced chicken
- 1 protein shake (300 calories or less)
- 1½ cups non-creamy soup (no potato soup or chowder) and a small green garden salad; try Easy Tomato Soup (see recipe, page 262)

Snack 3

Choose one of the following:

- 1 apple
- 1 pear
- 20 kale chips
- 1½ cups veggie juice (not from concentrate)
- 12 chocolate-covered almonds
- ½ cup edamame and sea salt to taste
- 1 baked medium tomato sprinkled with 2 teaspoons organic Parmesan cheese

Exercise

30 minutes of cardiovascular activity. You can do it all in one session or you can break it up into two different sessions. Choose a combination of the items below to fulfill your exercise requirement.

Gym Options

- 15 minutes of walking/running on treadmill
- 15 minutes on elliptical machine
- 15 minutes on stationary bicycle

- 15 minutes of swimming laps
- 15 minutes on stair climber
- 15 minutes of spinning
- 15 minutes of rowing machine
- 20 minutes of treadmill intervals

Non-gym Options

- 15 minutes of jogging outside
- 225 jump rope revolutions
- 15 minutes of brisk walking
- 15 minutes of walking up and down a staircase of at least 10 stairs. Walking up and down the staircase is considered 1 set (rest between sets as needed).
- 15 minutes of Zumba
- 15 minutes of riding bicycle outside
- 15 minutes of hiking
- 15 minutes of any other high-intensity cardio
- 15 minutes of alternating between running and walking. Run for 1 minute, then walk for 1 minute, then run again and walk again. Repeat the cycle for 15 minutes.

DAY 3

Meal 1

- 1 cup lemon water: Pour 8 ounces water, either hot or cold. Squeeze the juice from half a lemon directly into the water.
- 1 piece of fruit. This can be 1 banana, 1 apple, 1 pear, etc. It can also be ½ cup raspberries, blueberries, blackberries, or strawberries.

Choose one of the following. Your portion should be 1 cup cooked.

- 1 small bowl of oatmeal with optional 1% or 2% milk, fruit, and 1 teaspoon brown sugar
- 1 small bowl of Cream of Wheat or farina with optional 1% or 2% milk, fruit, and 1 teaspoon brown sugar
- 1 small bowl of grits with optional 1% or 2% milk, fruit, and 1 teaspoon brown sugar

Snack 1

Choose one of the following:

- Raw trail mix (1 cup raw nuts, sunflower or pumpkin seeds, and dried fruit)
- 4 dates stuffed with almonds (take out the pits and replace with a few almonds)
- ½ cup total of raisins, raw walnuts, and a pinch of sea salt (mix together)
- 3 tomato slices and fresh basil drizzled with olive oil
- ½ cucumber, sliced, sprinkled with a pinch of sea salt and fat-free vinaigrette dressing
- 1 cup unsweetened applesauce
- 10 cherries mixed with a handful of nuts (cashews, almonds, or walnuts)

- 8 baby carrots with 2 tablespoons hummus
- Ants on a log (2 celery sticks dabbed with 1 tablespoon raw nut butter and 1 tablespoon organic raisins)
- 1 piece of medium-size fruit
- Small beet or carrot salad
- 1 cup beet or carrot juice

Meal 2
Choose one of the following.
- 1 fruit smoothie (300 calories or less)
- 1 protein shake (300 calories or less). Try the Blustery Banana Shake (see recipe, page 289).
- 1½ cups soup (no potatoes, no cream). Good choices are chicken noodle, vegetable, lentil, chickpea, split pea, black bean, tomato bisque, etc. Be careful of sodium content! Try for low sodium: 140 mg or less per serving.

Snack 2
Choose one of the following:
- Raw trail mix (½ cup raw nuts, sunflower or pumpkin seeds, and dried fruit)
- 1 date stuffed with almonds (take out the pit and replace with a few almonds)
- ½ cup raisins, raw walnuts, and a pinch of sea salt (mix together)
- 3 tomato slices and fresh basil drizzled with olive oil
- ½ cucumber, sliced, sprinkled with a pinch of sea salt and fat-free vinaigrette dressing
- 1 cup unsweetened applesauce
- 10 cherries mixed with a handful of nuts (cashews, almonds, or walnuts)

- 8 baby carrots with 2 tablespoons hummus
- Ants on a log (2 celery sticks dabbed with 1 tablespoon raw nut butter and 1 tablespoon organic raisins)
- 1 piece of medium-size fruit
- Small beet or carrot salad
- 1 cup beet or carrot juice

Meal 3
Choose one of the following.
- 6-ounce piece of chicken (no skin, no frying) with ½ cup brown rice and 1 vegetable
- 6-ounce piece of fish (no frying) with ½ cup brown rice and 1 vegetable
- 6-ounce piece of turkey (no skin, no frying) with ½ cup brown rice and 1 vegetable
- 4 servings of vegetables with 1 cup brown rice
- Supreme Strip Steak (see recipe, page 275), with 2 servings of veggies

Snack 3
Choose one of the following:
- Raw trail mix (½ cup raw nuts, with sunflower or pumpkin seeds, and dried fruit)
- 2 dates stuffed with almonds (take out the pits and replace with a few almonds)
- ½ cup raisins, raw walnuts, and a pinch of sea salt (mix together)
- 3 tomato slices and fresh basil drizzled with olive oil
- ½ cucumber, sliced, sprinkled with a pinch of sea salt and fat-free vinaigrette dressing
- 1 cup unsweetened applesauce

- 10 cherries mixed with a handful of nuts (cashews, almonds, or walnuts)
- 8 baby carrots with 2 tablespoons hummus
- Ants on a log (2 celery sticks dabbed with 1 tablespoon raw nut butter and 1 tablespoon organic raisins)
- 1 piece of medium-size fruit
- Small beet or carrot salad
- 1 cup beet or carrot juice

Exercise
Rest day

| | | | | | | | | | | | | | | **DAY 4** | | | | | | | | | | | | | | | | |

Meal 1

- 1 cup lemon water: Pour 8 ounces water, either hot or cold. Squeeze the juice from half a lemon directly into the water.
- 1 cup raspberries, sliced strawberries, blueberries, or blackberries

Choose one of the following:
- 1 fruit smoothie (300 calories or less and no sugar added). Try the Sweet Kale-acious Smoothie (see recipe, page 286).
- 1 protein shake (300 calories or less and no sugar added)

Snack 1

- Any item 150 calories or less

Meal 2

Choose one of the following:
- 4 servings of vegetables. Remember, a serving is about the size of the average person's fist.
- Large green salad (all or any of the following: lettuce, 5 olives, 3 tablespoons shredded cheese, 5 cherry tomatoes, 2 tablespoons nuts, sliced cucumbers) with 2 tablespoons low-fat or fat-free vinaigrette-type dressing and 3 ounces sliced chicken or ½ cup beans if desired; no bacon bits and no croutons
- 1 protein shake (300 calories or less)

Snack 2

- Any item 150 calories or less

Meal 3

Choose one of the following:

- 1 bowl of soup (300 calories or less; no potatoes, no cream) with 2 servings of veggies
- 6-ounce piece of chicken (no skin, no frying) with 2 servings of veggies
- 6-ounce piece of fish (no frying) with 2 servings of veggies
- 6-ounce piece of turkey (no skin, no frying) with 2 servings of veggies
- 4 servings of veggies with 1 cup brown rice
- Honey Soy Glazed Salmon (see recipe, page 274), with 2 servings of veggies

Snack 3

- Any item 100 calories or less

Exercise

The exercises below do not have to be done in one session. You should fulfill these requirements over the course of the day. Use a wearable device or your smartphone to keep a tally of your step count for the day. Make sure you are using a set of stairs that has at least 10 steps and no more than 15.

- 12,000 steps throughout the day
- 15 sets of stairs (up and down is considered 1 set)

||||||||||||||| **DAY 5** |||||||||||||||||

Meal 1
- 1 cup lemon water: Pour 8 ounces water, either hot or cold. Squeeze the juice from half a lemon directly into the water.

Choose one of the following. Your portion should be 1 cup cooked.
- 1 small bowl of oatmeal with optional 1% or 2% milk, fruit, and 1 teaspoon brown sugar
- 1 small bowl of Cream of Wheat or farina with optional 1% or 2% milk, fruit, and 1 teaspoon brown sugar
- 1 small bowl of grits with optional 1% or 2% milk, fruit, and 1 teaspoon brown sugar
- Baked Apple Heaven (see recipe, page 255)

Snack 1
Choose one of the following:
- Raw trail mix (1 cup raw nuts, sunflower or pumpkin seeds, and dried fruit)
- 3 dates stuffed with almonds (take out the pits and replace with a few almonds)
- ½ cup raisins, raw walnuts, and a pinch of sea salt (mix together)
- 3 tomato slices and fresh basil drizzled with olive oil
- ½ cucumber, sliced, sprinkled with a pinch of sea salt and fat-free vinaigrette dressing
- 1 cup unsweetened applesauce
- 10 cherries mixed with a handful of nuts (cashews, almonds, or walnuts)
- 8 baby carrots with 2 tablespoons hummus

- Ants on a log (2 celery sticks dabbed with 1 tablespoon raw nut butter and 1 tablespoon organic raisins)
- 1 piece of medium-size fruit
- Small beet or carrot salad
- 1 cup beet or carrot juice

Meal 2

Choose one of the following. Your choice must be 200 calories or less.

- 1 fruit smoothie
- 1 protein shake
- 1 bowl of soup (no potatoes, no cream) with a small green garden salad. Good choices are chicken noodle, vegetable, lentil, chickpea, split pea, black bean, tomato bisque, etc. Try for low sodium: 140 mg or less per serving. Try the Luscious Pea Soup (see recipe, page 263).
- 6-ounce piece of grilled or baked chicken or fish with 2 servings of veggies

Snack 2

Choose one of the following:

- Raw trail mix (½ cup raw nuts, with sunflower or pumpkin seeds, and dried fruit)
- 1 date stuffed with almonds (take out the pit and replace with a few almonds)
- ½ cup raisins, raw walnuts, and a pinch of sea salt (mix together)
- 3 tomato slices and fresh basil drizzled with olive oil
- ½ cucumber, sliced, sprinkled with a pinch of sea salt and fat-free vinaigrette dressing
- 1 cup unsweetened applesauce
- 10 cherries mixed with a handful of nuts (cashews, almonds, or walnuts)

- 8 baby carrots with 2 tablespoons hummus
- Ants on a log (2 celery sticks dabbed with 1 tablespoon raw nut butter and 1 tablespoon organic raisins)
- 1 piece of medium-size fruit
- Small beet or carrot salad
- 1 cup beet or carrot juice

Meal 3

Choose one of the following:
- 6-ounce piece of chicken (no skin, no frying) with ½ cup brown rice and 1 serving of veggies
- 6-ounce piece of fish (no frying) with ½ cup brown rice and 1 serving of veggies
- 6-ounce piece of turkey (no skin, no frying) with ½ cup brown rice and 1 serving of veggies
- 4 servings of vegetables and 1 cup brown rice

Snack 3

Choose one of the following:
- Raw trail mix (½ cup raw nuts, with sunflower or pumpkin seeds, and dried fruit)
- 1 date stuffed with almonds (take out the pit and replace with a few almonds)
- ½ cup raisins, raw walnuts, and a pinch of sea salt (mix together)
- 3 tomato slices and fresh basil drizzled with olive oil
- ½ cucumber, sliced, sprinkled with a pinch of sea salt and fat-free vinaigrette dressing
- 1 cup unsweetened applesauce
- 10 cherries mixed with a handful of nuts (cashews, almonds, or walnuts)
- 8 baby carrots with 2 tablespoons hummus

- Ants on a log (2 celery sticks dabbed with 1 tablespoon raw nut butter and 1 tablespoon organic raisins)
- 1 piece of medium-size fruit
- Small beet or carrot salad
- 1 cup beet or carrot juice

Exercise

30 minutes of cardiovascular activity. You can do it all in one session or you can break it up into two different sessions. Choose a combination of the items below to fulfill your exercise requirement.

Gym Options

- 15 minutes walking/running on treadmill
- 15 minutes on elliptical machine
- 15 minutes on stationary bicycle
- 15 minutes of swimming laps
- 15 minutes on stair climber
- 15 minutes of spinning
- 15 minutes of rowing machine
- 20 minutes of treadmill intervals

Non-gym Options

- 15 minutes of jogging outside
- 225 jump rope revolutions
- 15 minutes of brisk walking
- 15 minutes of walking up and down a staircase of at least 10 stairs; walking up and down the staircase is considered 1 set (rest between sets as needed)
- 15 minutes of Zumba
- 15 minutes of riding bicycle outside
- 15 minutes of hiking

- 15 minutes of any other high-intensity cardio
- 15 minutes of alternating between running and walking. Run for 1 minute, then walk for 1 minute, then run again and walk again. Repeat the cycle for 15 minutes.

DAY 6

Meal 1
- 1 cup lemon water: Pour 8 ounces water, either hot or cold. Squeeze the juice from half a lemon directly into the water.

Choose one of the following:
- 1½ cups oatmeal with optional 1% or 2% milk, fruit, and 1 teaspoon brown sugar
- 2 egg whites *or* 1 egg-white omelet with diced veggies (made with 2 egg whites max) and 1 serving of fruit
- 1 small bowl of sugar-free cereal with fat-free, skim, or 1% or 2% milk and 1 serving of fruit
- 1 grilled cheese (2 slices of cheese 3½ inches square) on 100% whole-grain or 100% whole-wheat bread and 1 serving of fruit
- Gramma's Old-Fashioned Pancakes (see recipe, page 256)

Snack 1
- Any item 150 calories or less

Meal 2
Choose one of the following:
- 1 fruit smoothie (300 calories or less and no added sugar)
- 1 protein shake (300 calories or less and no added sugar)
- 1 veggie shake (300 calories or less and no added sugar)
- 1½ cups soup (no potatoes, no cream sauces, no meat). Good choices are vegetable, lentil, chickpea, split pea, black bean, tomato bisque, etc. Be careful of sodium content! Try for low sodium: 140 mg or less per serving. Try the Smooth Lentil Soup (see recipe, page 264).

Snack 2

- Any item 150 calories or less

Meal 3

Choose one of the following:

- 1½ cups soup (no potatoes, no cream) with a small green garden salad. Good choices are vegetable, lentil, chickpea, split pea, black bean, tomato bisque, etc. Be careful of sodium content! Try for low sodium: 140 mg or less per serving.
- 6-ounce veggie or turkey burger without the bun with a small green garden salad

Snack 3

- Any item 150 calories or less

Exercise

Rest day

DAY 7

Meal 1

- 1 cup lemon water: Pour 8 ounces water, either hot or cold. Squeeze the juice from half a lemon directly into the water.

Choose one of the following:

- 1 fruit smoothie (300 calories or less with no added sugar)
- 1 protein shake (300 calories or less with no added sugar)
- 1 veggie shake (300 calories or less with no added sugar)
- 6 ounces low-fat or fat-free Greek yogurt; add fresh fruit and 1 tablespoon granola if desired

Snack 1

Choose one of the following:

- Raw trail mix (½ cup raw nuts, with sunflower or pumpkin seeds, and dried fruit)
- 2 dates stuffed with almonds (take out the pits and replace with a few almonds)
- ½ cup raisins, raw walnuts, and a pinch of sea salt (mix together)
- 3 tomato slices and fresh basil drizzled with olive oil
- ½ cucumber, sliced, sprinkled with a pinch of sea salt and fat-free vinaigrette dressing
- 1 cup unsweetened applesauce
- 10 cherries mixed with a handful of nuts (cashews, almonds, or walnuts)
- 8 baby carrots with 2 tablespoons hummus

- Ants on a log (2 celery sticks dabbed with 1 tablespoon raw nut butter and 1 tablespoon organic raisins)
- 1 piece of medium-size fruit
- Small beet or carrot salad
- 1 cup beet or carrot juice
- 20 almonds
- Small fruit cup
- 8 dried apricot halves
- 3 tablespoons sunflower seeds

Meal 2

Choose one of the following:

- Turkey sandwich on 100% whole-grain or 100% whole-wheat toast with lettuce, cheese, and tomato optional and your choice of 1 tablespoon spread like mayonnaise or mustard or dressing and a small salad
- Chicken sandwich on 100% whole-grain or 100% whole-wheat toast with lettuce, cheese, and tomato optional and your choice of 1 tablespoon spread like mayonnaise or mustard or dressing and a small salad
- 1½ cups soup (no potatoes, no cream) with a small salad. Good choices are vegetable, lentil, chickpea, split pea, black bean, tomato bisque, etc. Be careful of sodium content. Try for low sodium: 140 mg or less per serving.
- Greek Energy Bowl (see recipe, page 260)

Snack 2

Choose one of the following:

- Raw trail mix (½ cup raw nuts, sunflower or pumpkin seeds, and dried fruit)
- 1 date stuffed with almonds (take out the pit and replace it with a few almonds)

- ½ cup raisins, raw walnuts, and a pinch of sea salt (mix together)
- 3 tomato slices and fresh basil drizzled with olive oil
- ½ cucumber, sliced, sprinkled with a pinch of sea salt and fat-free vinaigrette dressing
- 1 cup unsweetened applesauce
- 10 cherries mixed with a handful of nuts (cashews, almonds, or walnuts)
- 8 baby carrots with 2 tablespoons hummus
- Ants on a log (2 celery sticks dabbed with 1 tablespoon raw nut butter and 1 tablespoon organic raisins)
- 1 piece of medium-size fruit
- Small beet or carrot salad
- 1 cup beet or carrot juice
- 20 almonds
- Small fruit cup
- 8 dried apricot halves
- 2 tablespoons sunflower seeds

Meal 3

Choose one of the following:
- 6-ounce piece of skinless chicken breast grilled or baked with ½ cup brown rice and 2 servings of veggies
- 6-ounce piece of fish (no frying) with ½ cup brown rice and 2 servings of veggies
- 6-ounce piece of turkey (no skin, no frying) with ½ cup brown rice and 2 servings of veggies
- Beef Burrito Bowl (see recipe, page 268)
- Large green salad (all or any of the following: lettuce, 5 olives, 3 tablespoons shredded cheese, 5 cherry tomatoes, 2 tablespoons nuts, sliced cucumbers) with 2 tablespoons

low-fat or fat-free vinaigrette-type dressing and 3 ounces sliced chicken or ½ cup beans if desired

Snack 3

Choose one of the following:

- Raw trail mix (½ cup raw nuts, sunflower or pumpkin seeds, and dried fruit)
- 1 date stuffed with almonds (take out the pit and replace with a few almonds)
- ½ cup raisins, raw walnuts, and a pinch of sea salt (mix together)
- 3 tomato slices and fresh basil drizzled with olive oil
- ½ cucumber, sliced, sprinkled with a pinch of sea salt and fat-free vinaigrette dressing
- 1 cup unsweetened applesauce
- 10 cherries mixed with 10 nuts (cashews, almonds, or walnuts)
- 8 baby carrots with 2 tablespoons hummus
- Ants on a log (2 celery sticks dabbed with 1 tablespoon raw nut butter and 1 tablespoon organic raisins)
- 1 piece of medium-size fruit
- Small beet or carrot salad
- 1 cup beet or carrot juice
- 20 almonds
- Small fruit cup
- 8 dried apricot halves
- 1 tablespoon sunflower seeds

Exercise

The exercises below do not have to be done in one session. You should fulfill these requirements over the course of the day. Use a wearable device or your smartphone to keep a tally of your step count for the day. Make sure you are using a set of stairs that has at least 10 steps and no more than 15.

- 12,000 steps throughout the day
- 15 sets of stairs (up and down is considered 1 set)

4

Week 2:

Turn Up

NOW THAT YOU ARE IN THE SECOND WEEK OF THE PLAN, it's time to turn up the burn a little. Each week builds on the previous week, so it's important to continue making progress. I never expect or mandate that you perform perfectly on the plan, but I simply ask that you do your best and continue to improve. After the previous seven days of eating differently on a new schedule, your body should now be reasonably acclimated to this style of intermittent fasting and clean eating. This second week is similar to the first, but there are some differences in calorie counts, meal choices, snacks, and exercises. Follow the guidelines as closely as possible and make good decisions. Spend a few minutes planning what you'll eat for the week and do your best to make sure you have these foods in the house or access to them if you're not going to be home. Proper preparation prevents poor performance.

Guidelines

- Continue to follow the fasting and feeding windows from week 1, but make sure you eat your first meal no earlier than two hours after getting up, and make sure your last meal does not occur within two hours of going to bed.

For example, if you get up at 6 A.M., don't eat until 8 A.M. If you go to sleep at 10 P.M., then your last meal must be before 8 P.M.

- You DO NOT have to eat all of the food that's listed. Eat enough to satiate. Eat slowly and mindfully enough that you can not only taste and enjoy your meals and snacks, but notice your body's cues that you are full. Don't eat until you're so full that you "can't eat another bite."

- Do your best to fulfill the exercise requirements for the day. You can always break up the exercise into two sessions. The key is that when you are exercising, you are actually exercising. Don't include your breaks in the exercise time.

- Beverages: You can have fresh juice (1 cup per day), herbal tea (unsweetened), unlimited plain water (still or fizzy), or water with freshly squeezed citrus like lemon or lime, 1 cup freshly squeezed lemonade per day, 2 cups 1% or 2% milk (soy, low-fat, skim, reduced-fat, coconut); 2 cups coffee per day (each coffee must be 50 calories or less).

- If a sandwich calls for cheese, note that it should be 1 slice of cheese of your choice and the size should be approximately 3½ inches square, which is the typical size of packaged cheese.

- NO white bread (100% whole-grain or 100% whole-wheat bread allowed).

- NO products made with white flour.

- NO white pasta (except in the case of chicken noodle soup).

- NO soda (regular or diet).

- NO alcohol.

- NO donuts, cake, brownies, pastries, muffins.
- NO creamy salad dressings.
- NO white potatoes.
- NO frying.

DAY 1

Meal 1

- 1 cup lemon water: Pour 8 ounces water, either hot or cold. Squeeze the juice from half a small lemon directly into the water. Add 2 tablespoons ground flaxseeds or flaxseed oil. Mix well and drink. You can also add the flaxseed to other beverages, or yogurt or cereal.

Choose one of the following:
- 1 fruit smoothie (300 calories or less; no sugar added)
- 1 protein shake (300 calories or less; no sugar added)
- 2 scrambled whole eggs (diced veggies and 3 tablespoons shredded cheese or 1 slice of cheese 3½ inches square optional; a little butter or cooking spray allowed)

Snack 1

- Any item 150 calories or less

Meal 2

Choose one of the following:
- 3 servings of vegetables with 1 cup brown rice. A serving is about the size of the average person's fist.
- Large green salad (all or any: lettuce, 5 olives, 3 tablespoons shredded cheese, 5 cherry tomatoes, 2 tablespoons nuts, sliced cucumbers) with 2 tablespoons low-fat or fat-free vinaigrette-type dressing and 3 ounces sliced chicken or ½ cup beans if desired
- 1 protein shake (300 calories or less) with a small green garden salad

Snack 2

- Any item 150 calories or less

Meal 3

Choose one of the following:

- 1 bowl of soup (300 calories or less; no potatoes, no cream) with 2 servings of veggies
- 6-ounce piece of chicken (no skin, no frying) with 2 servings of veggies
- 6-ounce piece of fish (no frying) with 2 servings of veggies
- 6-ounce piece of turkey (no skin, no frying) with 2 servings of veggies
- 4 servings of veggies

Snack 3

- Any item 150 calories or less

Exercise

- 12,000 steps to be completed throughout the day
- 15 sets of stairs (up and down is considered 1 set)

| | | | | | | | | | | | | | | **DAY 2** | | | | | | | | | | | | | | |

Meal 1

- 1 cup lemon water: Pour 8 ounces water, either hot or cold. Squeeze the juice from half a small lemon directly into the water. Add 2 tablespoons ground flaxseeds or flaxseed oil. Mix well and drink. You can also add the flaxseed to other beverages, or yogurt or cereal.

Choose one of the following:

- 1 cup cooked oatmeal (optional: 1% or 2% milk, raisins or blueberries, 1 teaspoon brown sugar)
- 1 cup Cream of Wheat or farina (optional: 1% or 2% milk, fruit, and 1 teaspoon sugar)
- 1 cup cold cereal (7 g or less sugar) with 1% or 2% milk with a serving of fruit

Snack 1

- Any item 150 calories or less

Meal 2

Choose one of the following:

- 1 protein shake (300 calories or less; no sugar added)
- 1 fruit smoothie (300 calories or less; no sugar added)
- 1 cup soup (no potatoes, no heavy cream) with a small garden salad. Good choices: chicken noodle, vegetable, lentil, chickpea, split pea, black bean, tomato basil, minestrone. Try for low sodium: 140 mg or less per serving.
- Chicken sandwich on 100% whole-grain or 100% whole-wheat toast with lettuce, 1 slice of cheese 3½ inches square, and tomato optional and your choice of 1 tablespoon spread like mayonnaise or mustard or dressing and a small salad

Snack 2

- Any item 150 calories or less

Meal 3

- Large green garden salad (3 cups greens) with 2½ ounces sliced chicken. You may include a few olives, shredded carrots, sliced cucumbers, and ½ sliced tomato or 5 grape tomatoes. Only 2 tablespoons fat-free or low-fat vinaigrette-type dressing (no bacon bits, no croutons).
- 1 cup whole-grain or chickpea pasta in a meatless tomato sauce with 1 serving of veggies mixed into the pasta
- 1 veggie or turkey burger on 100% whole-grain bun with lettuce, 1 slice of cheese, and tomato, and 1 tablespoon your choice of spread

Snack 3

- Any item 150 calories or less

Exercise

Amount of exercise today: minimum 40 minutes. If you want to do more, all the better! Work as hard as you can! The key is to avoid doing steady-state exercise such as walking on the treadmill at the same speed and same incline for a period of time. Instead, try to vary your speed, your incline, the distances you cover. The goal here is to do high-intensity interval training.

Choose two of the cardiovascular exercises below, for a total of 40 minutes of exercise.

Gym Options

- 20 minutes of walking/running on treadmill
- 20 minutes on elliptical machine
- 20 minutes on stationary bicycle
- 20 minutes of swimming laps
- 20 minutes on stair climber

- 20 minutes of spinning
- 20 minutes of rowing machine
- 20 minutes of treadmill intervals

Non-gym Options

- 20 minutes of jogging outside
- 225 jump rope revolutions
- 20 minutes of brisk walking
- 20 minutes of walking up and down a staircase of at least 10 stairs; walking up and down the staircase is considered 1 set (rest between sets as needed)
- 20 minutes of Zumba
- 20 minutes of riding bicycle outside
- 20 minutes of hiking
- 20 minutes of any other high-intensity cardio
- 20 minutes of alternating between running and walking. Run for 1 minute, then walk for 1 minute, then run again and walk again. Repeat the cycle for 20 minutes.

| | | | | | | | | | | | | | | **DAY 3** | | | | | | | | | | | | | |

Meal 1

- 1 cup lemon water: Pour 8 ounces water, either hot or cold. Squeeze the juice from half a small lemon directly into the water. Add 2 tablespoons ground flaxseeds or flaxseed oil. Mix well and drink. You can also add the flaxseed to other beverages, or yogurt or cereal.

Choose one of the following:

- Smoothie (300 calories or less; no sugar added)
- Protein shake (300 calories or less; no sugar added)
- 1 cup steel-cut oats with sliced apples and walnuts, 1% or 2% milk and 1 teaspoon brown sugar optional

Snack 1

- Any item 150 calories or less

Meal 2

Choose one of the following:

- 2 cups total of tomato, cucumber, onion, black or white bean salad with 3 tablespoons balsamic vinaigrette
- Lettuce, cheese, tomato sandwich on 100% whole-grain or whole-wheat with choice of spread
- 1 cup soup (no potatoes, no cream) with a small garden salad. Good choices: chicken noodle, vegetable, lentil, chickpea, split pea, black bean, tomato basil, minestrone. Try for low sodium: 140 mg or less per serving.

Snack 2

- Any item 150 calories or less

Meal 3

Choose one of the following:

- Cauliflower and brown rice stuffed peppers (enough to fill both halves of a small pepper)
- Portobello mushroom steaks: First marinate in spices and soy sauce or balsamic vinaigrette, then cook in a touch of olive oil and salt and pepper to taste.
- 6-ounce piece of grilled or baked fish with 2 servings of vegetables

Snack 3

- Any item 150 calories or less

Exercise

Rest day

| | | | | | | | | | | | | | | | | **DAY 4** | | | | | | | | | | | | | | | |

Meal 1

- 1 cup lemon water: Pour 8 ounces water, either hot or cold. Squeeze the juice from half a small lemon directly into the water. Add 2 tablespoons ground flaxseeds or flaxseed oil. Mix well and drink. You can also add the flaxseed to other beverages, or yogurt or cereal.

Choose one of the following:

- 6 ounces low-fat, plain Greek yogurt with fresh fruit
- 1 egg-white omelet (made with 2 egg whites or ½ cup Egg Beaters; a little butter or cooking spray allowed) with 1 serving of fruit
- 1 cup cold cereal (7 g or less sugar) with 1% or 2% milk with 1 serving of fruit

Optional: 1 piece of 100% whole-grain or 100% whole-wheat toast with any of the above options you choose

Snack 1

- Any item 150 calories or less

Meal 2

Choose one of the following. Your choice must not exceed 300 calories if you choose the smoothie or shake; no sugar added.

- 1 protein shake (300 calories or less; no sugar added)
- 1 fruit smoothie (300 calories or less; no sugar added)
- 1 cup soup (no potatoes, no cream). Good choices are chicken noodle, vegetable, lentil, chickpea, split pea, black bean, tomato basil, minestrone. Always be careful of sodium content! Try for low sodium: 140 mg or less per serving.

- Large green salad (all or any of the following: lettuce, 5 olives, 3 tablespoons shredded cheese, 5 cherry tomatoes, 2 tablespoons nuts, sliced cucumbers) with 2 tablespoons low-fat or fat-free vinaigrette-type dressing and 3 ounces sliced chicken or ½ cup beans if desired

Snack 2
- Any item 150 calories or less

Meal 3
Choose one of the following:
- 1 cup brown rice with 1 cup cooked beans, chickpeas, or lentils (no baked beans) and 1 serving of vegetables
- Large green salad (all or any of the following: lettuce, 5 olives, 3 tablespoons shredded cheese, 5 cherry tomatoes, 2 tablespoons nuts, sliced cucumbers) with 2 tablespoons low-fat or fat-free vinaigrette-type dressing and 3 ounces sliced chicken or ½ cup beans if desired; no bacon bits and no croutons

Snack 3
- Any item 150 calories or less

Exercise
- 14,000 steps throughout the day. Use your wearable device or smartphone to keep track.
- 15 sets of stairs (up and down is considered 1 set).

| | | | | | | | | | | | | | | | | **DAY 5** | | | | | | | | | | | | | | | | | |

Meal 1

- 1 cup lemon water: Pour 8 oz water, hot or cold, and squeeze in half a small lemon. Add 2 tablespoons ground flaxseeds or flaxseed oil. Mix well and drink. You can add the flaxseed to other beverages, yogurt, or cereal.

Choose one of the following:

- 1 cup cooked oatmeal with optional 1% or 2% milk or unsweetened soy or almond milk, raisins or blueberries, 1 teaspoon brown sugar
- 1 cup Cream of Wheat or farina with optional 1% or 2% milk, fruit, and 1 teaspoon brown sugar
- 6 ounces low-fat or fat-free plain Greek yogurt with fresh fruit

Snack 1

- Any item 150 calories or less

Meal 2

Choose one of the following:

- 3 servings of vegetables with 1 cup brown rice
- 5-ounce turkey or veggie burger on 100% whole-grain bread (1 slice of cheese 3½ inches square, tomato, lettuce optional)
- 1½ cups soup (no potatoes, no cream) with a small green garden salad. Good choices are chicken noodle, vegetable, lentil, chickpea, split pea, black bean, tomato basil, minestrone. Always be careful of sodium content! Try for low sodium: 140 mg or less per serving.

Snack 2

- Any item 150 calories or less

Meal 3

Choose one of the following:
- 6-ounce piece of turkey, chicken, or fish (grilled or baked, no skin, not fried) with 2 servings of veggies
- Vegetarian plate of 4 steamed vegetables and 1 cup brown rice

Snack 3

- Any item 150 calories or less

Exercise

40 minutes. Remember, you can always break up the workout. If you don't have time to do it all at once, you can do 20 minutes now and 20 later, or whatever combination works for you. Choose a combination of the items below to fulfill your exercise requirement:

Gym Options

- 20 minutes of walking/running on treadmill
- 20 minutes on elliptical machine
- 20 minutes on stationary bicycle
- 20 minutes of swimming laps
- 20 minutes on stair climber
- 20 minutes of spinning
- 20 minutes of rowing machine
- 20 minutes of treadmill intervals

Non-gym Options

- 15 minutes of jogging outside
- 225 jump rope revolutions
- 15 minutes of brisk walking
- 15 minutes of walking up and down a staircase of at least 10 stairs; walking up and down the staircase is considered 1 set (rest between sets as needed)

- 15 minutes of Zumba
- 15 minutes of riding bicycle outside
- 15 minutes of hiking
- 15 minutes of any other high-intensity cardio
- 15 minutes of alternating between running and walking. Run for 1 minute, then walk for 1 minute, then run again and walk again. Repeat the cycle for 15 minutes.

| | | | | | | | | | | | | | | **DAY 6** | | | | | | | | | | | | | | | | | |

Meal 1

- 1 cup lemon water: Pour 8 ounces water, either hot or cold. Squeeze the juice from half a small lemon directly into the water. Add 2 tablespoons ground flaxseeds or flaxseed oil. Mix well and drink. You can also add the flaxseed to other beverages, or yogurt or cereal.

Choose one of the following:
- 1 grilled cheese sandwich on 100% whole-grain or 100% whole-wheat bread (2 slices of cheese 3½ inches square)
- 1 cup low-fat or nonfat plain Greek yogurt with ⅓ cup granola or muesli and ¼ cup berries

Snack 1

- Any item 150 calories or less

Meal 2

Choose one of the following:
- Black bean wrap with avocados, diced tomatoes, lettuce, and brown rice on 100% whole-grain tortilla
- Large green salad (all or any: lettuce 5 olives, 3 tablespoons shredded cheese, 5 cherry tomatoes, 2 tablespoons nuts, sliced cucumbers) with 2 tablespoons low-fat or fat-free vinaigrette-type dressing and 3 ounces sliced chicken or ½ cup beans if desired; no bacon bits and no croutons

Snack 2

- Any item 150 calories or less

Meal 3

Choose one of the following:

- One serving each of 4 different steamed or raw vegetables with 1 cup brown rice
- 1 cup total of whole-grain spaghetti with optional diced zucchini, squash, peppers, tomatoes, and/or broccoli in a marinara or lemon-wine sauce

Snack 3
- Any item 150 calories or less

Exercise
Rest day

| | | | | | | | | | | | | | | | **DAY 7** | | | | | | | | | | | | | | | | |

Meal 1

- 1 cup lemon water: Pour 8 ounces water, either hot or cold, and squeeze in half a small lemon. Add 2 tablespoons ground flaxseeds or flaxseed oil. Mix well and drink. You can also add the flaxseed to yogurt or cereal.

Choose one of the following:
- 1 fruit smoothie (300 calories or less; no sugar added)
- 1 protein shake (300 calories or less; no sugar added)
- 1 cup cold cereal (7 g or less sugar) with 1% or 2% milk with 1 serving of fruit
- 1 egg-white omelet (2 egg whites or ½ cup Egg Beaters, ¼ cup cheese; a little butter or cooking spray is allowed)

Snack 1

- Any item 150 calories or less

Meal 2

- 1½ cups soup (no potatoes, no cream). Good choices are chicken noodle, vegetable, lentil, chickpea, split pea, black bean, tomato basil, minestrone. Try for low sodium: 140 mg or less per serving.

- Large green salad (all or any: lettuce, 5 olives, 3 tablespoons shredded cheese, 5 cherry tomatoes, 2 tablespoons nuts, sliced cucumbers) with 2 tablespoons low-fat or fat-free vinaigrette dressing and 3 ounces sliced chicken or ½ cup beans if desired; no bacon or croutons

Snack 2

- Any item 150 calories or less

Meal 3

Choose one of the following:

- 6-ounce piece of grilled or baked chicken breast (no skin) with 2 servings of vegetables
- 6-ounce piece of turkey with 2 servings of vegetables
- 6-ounce piece of grilled or baked fish with 2 servings of vegetables

Snack 3

- Any item 150 calories or less

Exercise

30 minutes. Choose a combination of the items below to fulfill your exercise requirement:

Gym Options

- 15 minutes of walking/running on treadmill
- 15 minutes on elliptical machine
- 15 minutes on stationary bicycle
- 15 minutes of swimming laps
- 15 minutes on stair climber
- 15 minutes of spinning
- 15 minutes of rowing machine
- 20 minutes of treadmill intervals

Non-gym Options

- 15 minutes of jogging outside
- 225 jump rope revolutions
- 15 minutes of brisk walking
- 15 minutes of walking up and down a staircase of at least 10 stairs; walking up and down the staircase is considered 1 set (rest between sets as needed)
- 15 minutes of Zumba

- 15 minutes of riding bicycle outside
- 15 minutes of hiking
- 15 minutes of any other high-intensity cardio
- 15 minutes of alternating between running and walking. Run for 1 minute, then walk for 1 minute, then run again and walk again. Repeat the cycle for 15 minutes.

5

Week 3:
Jigsaw Week #1

THIS IS A VERY DIFFERENT WEEK. BELOW YOU WILL FIND A new group of breakfasts, meals, lunches, and dinners. You choose what you want from each group for the day, but it's one breakfast, one lunch, and one dinner per day. The meals and snacks are provided to you like the pieces of a puzzle and you will assemble them like a jigsaw. You will also be allowed three snacks. These snacks MUST come from the snack list below, so check it out right away and go and get the ingredients you might need. You can eat the meals in any order you want and the snacks whenever you want, but I highly suggest you eat the snacks between the meals and not consecutively. You can only have the same breakfast, lunch, or dinner two days in a row, maximum. For example, you can have eggs two days in a row for breakfast, but you must have something else on the third day. Varying your foods is important for optimal success on the plan. This is an important week, because after two very structured weeks, you get a chance to put all that you've learned to the test and start configuring your own days and making your own decisions. Think hard, make good choices, and have confidence that you can do this!

This week will also see a change in your IF schedule. Go from a 12:12 to 14:10—a 14-hour fasting window and a 10-hour feeding window. Same rules apply as far as the 50-calorie allowance with beverages in your fasting window. To get the most out of turning on your body's fat-burning mode and increasing your energy demand, try to do most if not all of your exercise during your fasting window and try to wait at least two hours after you're done exercising to eat. For example, if you decide to exercise at 7 A.M., make sure you don't start your feeding window until 9 A.M. Another option is at night. If your feeding window ends at 8 P.M., try doing something physically exertive after your feeding window has ended and before you go to sleep. It might only be fifteen minutes of physical activity, but don't minimize the value of those fifteen minutes, as they can have a positive impact and help get you closer to your goals. Below are some of the guidelines you should follow this week.

Guidelines

- Wait at least two hours after you wake up before eating your breakfast. You can't have anything to eat within two hours of going to sleep. (Keep these guidelines in mind when setting your fasting/feeding windows.)

- You are allowed a glass of wine every other day this week. You can substitute a lite beer for the wine, but you can't have both on the same day—only one drink allowed on your drink day.

- You must drink 1 full cup of plain water before starting to eat each meal. You can add lemon or lime if you prefer.

- You must choose your snacks from those that are listed below. These snacks are selected because most of them tend to be high in nutritional density, but lower in calories. This means you're getting more bang for your caloric buck.

- Your beverage guidelines for what you can consume during your feeding window are as follows: you can have fresh juice (1 cup per day), unlimited herbal tea (unsweetened), unlimited plain water (still or fizzy), or water with freshly squeezed citrus like lemon or lime

- You can have some or all of the following: 1 cup freshly squeezed lemonade per day, 2 cups 1% or 2% milk (soy, low-fat, skim, reduced-fat, coconut); 2 cups coffee per day (each coffee must be 50 calories or less).
- If a sandwich calls for cheese, it should be 1 slice cheese of your choice. The size should be about 3½ inches square (the typical size of packaged cheese).
- NO white bread (100% whole-grain or 100% whole-wheat bread allowed) or products made with white flour.
- NO soda (regular or diet).
- NO donuts, cake, brownies, pastries, muffins.
- NO creamy salad dressings or sauces.
- NO white potatoes.
- NO frying.

Breakfast Options

For your breakfast options, choose from the list below. You can have only one of these options per day. Try to vary your choices to prevent food boredom and create more excitement in your culinary experience.

- Red pepper and scallion egg scramble (see omelet recipe on page 91)
- 1 cup cooked oatmeal with blueberries or bananas
- 2 scrambled eggs with 3 tablespoons shredded cheese

or 1 slice of cheese 3½ inches square and diced veggies and 2 slices of bacon

- 3 scrambled egg whites with ham and mushrooms
- Breakfast smoothie (350 calories or less). Try the Tropical Dash Smoothie (see recipe, page 285).
- 1 cup cold cereal (7 grams or less sugar) with 1% or 2% milk
- 8-ounce yogurt parfait made with plain Greek yogurt, ¼ cup granola, and fruit of your choice
- One slice of avocado toast (smashed avocado and salt and pepper to taste spread on toast) with 1 piece of fruit
- Chocolate pudding: In a saucepan, stir together 2 teaspoons organic honey, 1 tablespoon cocoa powder, 1 tablespoon cornstarch, and ⅛ teaspoon salt. Place over medium heat and stir in ⅓ cup unsweetened almond milk or whole milk. Bring to a boil and stir constantly while cooking, until mixture thickens. Remove from heat and stir in ½ tablespoon room-temperature butter and 1 teaspoon vanilla extract. Scoop into a small jar or bowl and refrigerate for at least 5 hours.
- Avocado and smoked salmon toast (1 toasted slice of 100% whole-grain or whole-wheat bread, ½ small avocado smashed in a bowl with a pinch of cayenne pepper, 2 tablespoons fresh lemon juice, 2 tablespoons low-fat or fat-free plain Greek yogurt, 3 ounces smoked salmon, and cucumber slices as a topping, salt and pepper to taste)
- 1 cup Cream of Wheat or farina with a side of fruit
- Egg and cheese muffin (1 scrambled egg with cheese and veggies on a toasted 100% whole-grain or 100% whole-wheat English muffin)
- Citrus salad: Slice ½ grapefruit and ½ orange into rounds

and arrange on a plate. Scoop 2 tablespoons low-fat or
fat-free plain Greek yogurt on top and drizzle with
2 teaspoons organic honey.

- Omelet with 3 tablespoons shredded cheese (or 1 slice of
cheese 3½ inches square); options: mushrooms, spinach,
peppers, and tomatoes
- 2 pancakes (5 inches in diameter) with 1 slice of bacon
and 1 teaspoon 100% pure maple syrup. Try Gramma's
Old-Fashioned Pancakes (see recipe, page 256).

Lunch Options

For your lunch options, choose from the list below. You can have
only one of these options per day. Try to vary your choices to prevent food boredom and create more excitement in your culinary
experience. Adding vegetables to any of the dishes, if not already
prescribed, is always an acceptable modification.

- Whole-wheat pasta with edamame pesto sauce (see recipe,
page 272)
- Tuna salad sandwich with lettuce on 100% whole-grain or
100% whole-wheat bread: Drain two 5-ounce cans water-
packed tuna and combine with 3 tablespoons mayonnaise,
1 finely diced celery rib, ¼ cup finely diced small red
onion, 1 tablespoon fresh lemon juice, 1 tablespoon pickle
relish, and salt and pepper to taste.
- Greek Energy Bowl (see recipe, page 260)
- Chicken salad sandwich on 100% whole-grain or 100%
whole-wheat bread
- 5-ounce veggie burger on 100% whole-grain or
100% whole-wheat bread with a small green garden
salad

- Turkey sandwich with lettuce, tomato, and cheese (1 slice 3½ inches square), with 1 tablespoon mustard or mayo on 100% whole-grain or 100% whole-wheat bread

- Chicken sandwich with lettuce, tomato, and cheese (1 slice 3½ inches square), with 1 tablespoon mayo on 100% whole-grain or 100% whole-wheat bread

- Large green garden salad (3 cups greens) with 2½ ounces sliced chicken. You may include a few olives, shredded carrots, sliced cucumbers, and ½ sliced tomato or 5 grape tomatoes. Only 2 tablespoons fat-free or low-fat vinaigrette-type dressing; no bacon bits and no croutons.

- 1½ cups soup (no potatoes, no cream). Good choices are chicken noodle, vegetable, lentil, chickpea, split pea, black bean, tomato bisque, etc. Be careful of sodium content! Try for low sodium: 140 mg or less per serving.

- 3 servings of vegetables with 1 cup brown rice

- 1 protein shake (350 calories or less)

- Vegetarian Mediterranean wrap: Take a whole-wheat tortilla and spread hummus on it, then top with a small sliced tomato, 3 chopped green or black olives, 1 tablespoon feta cheese, and ½ tablespoon fresh lemon juice.

- Sprightly Watermelon Feta Salad (see recipe, page 267)

- 6-ounce beef burger on a 100% whole-grain or 100% whole-wheat bun with lettuce, cheese, and tomato optional, along with a small green garden salad

- Burrito bowl (2 cups brown rice, beans of your choice, tomato, avocado, onion, shredded lettuce)

- Veggie and hummus sandwich on 100% whole-grain or 100% whole-wheat bread

- Greek salad with pita: Combine 2 cups kale or romaine leaves, ¼ cup black beans, ¼ cup chickpeas, 2 tablespoons

diced red onion, 1 tablespoon cilantro, juice of 1 lime,
½ whole-grain pita cut into slices, ¼ cup sweet corn, and
optional ½ cup diced chicken.

- Toasty Tuna Melt (see recipe, page 259) with a small salad
- Ham sandwich on 100% whole-grain or 100% whole-
  wheat bread with lettuce, tomato, 1 slice of cheese (3½
  inches square), and 1 tablespoon mustard or mayo (only
  2 thin slices of ham).

Dinner Options

For your dinner options, choose from the list below. You can have
only one of these options per day. Try to vary your choices to prevent food boredom and create more excitement in your culinary
experience. Adding vegetables to any of the dishes, if not already
prescribed, is always an acceptable modification.

- 6-ounce piece of chicken (no skin, no frying) with
  2 servings of vegetables
- 6-ounce piece of fish (no frying) with 2 servings of
  vegetables
- 6-ounce piece of turkey (no skin, no frying) with
  2 servings of vegetables
- Chicken burger on a 100% whole-wheat bun with lettuce,
  tomato, and cheese optional and a small green garden
  salad
- 4 servings of steamed vegetables and 1 cup brown rice
- 6-ounce turkey burger with 2 servings of vegetables
- 1 cup whole-grain or whole-wheat pasta with sliced
  chicken or fish and veggies (in a tomato-based or wine
  sauce—NO cream)

- Chicken or beef stew with quinoa or brown rice and beans
- 1 large bell pepper stuffed with ground beef and cheese: Cook ground beef in extra-virgin olive oil with ¼ cup chopped onions, diced tomatoes, 3 tablespoons shredded cheese, 1 minced clove garlic, ½ teaspoon dried oregano, salt and pepper to taste.
- Cheesy Chicken Quesadilla with 1 serving of vegetables and brown rice (see recipe, page 277)
- 6-ounce tuna steak with 1 small sweet potato and 1 serving of green vegetables
- 1½ cups vegetarian chili soup (1 tablespoon extra-virgin olive oil, 2 minced cloves garlic, 1 chopped small yellow onion, 1 red pepper cut into small chunks, 1 cup sweet corn, ½ tablespoon mild chili powder, 1 teaspoon ground cumin, 1 teaspoon dried oregano, ½ tablespoon balsamic vinegar, ½ tablespoon brown sugar, ½ cup diced tomatoes, 1 cup black beans, ½ cup red beans, 1 cup low-sodium vegetable stock; makes 3 servings)
- Beef stir-fry with brown rice, broccoli, corn, and diced peppers
- 6-ounce lean steak with 2 servings of veggies
- Spaghetti and meatballs made with whole-grain, whole-wheat, or chickpea pasta and 3 meatballs

Snacks
- 2 hard-boiled eggs with seasoning
- Tomato and mozzarella: Cut a 1-ounce slice of fresh mozzarella into small cubes, then place in a small bowl with 10 halved cherry tomatoes and 1 to 2 teaspoons chopped fresh basil. Drizzle with 1 tablespoon balsamic glaze or balsamic vinaigrette.
- 1 piece of fruit

- 2 clementines with 20 pistachios
- 20 raw almonds
- 45 pistachios
- 15 cucumber slices and 2 tablespoons peanut butter
- 6 ounces low-fat plain Greek yogurt
- 15 cashews
- 25 dry-roasted peanuts
- Yogurt-dipped strawberries: Take 1 cup rinsed whole strawberries and individually dip them about three-fourths of the way up in ⅓ cup vanilla low-fat Greek yogurt. Place on a parchment paper–lined baking sheet to freeze, then store in an airtight container in the freezer.
- 2 tablespoons sunflower or pumpkin seeds
- 1 medium banana and 1 tablespoon cottage cheese
- 2 stalks celery and 4 tablespoons hummus
- 8 baby carrot sticks (or 20 cucumber slices) and 4 tablespoons hummus
- 1 small baked sweet potato with 2 tablespoons fat-free sour cream or a little butter
- 2 cups air-popped popcorn with small amount of salt
- 1 fat-free chocolate or vanilla pudding
- 1½ cups sugar snap peas
- 1 hard-boiled egg (lightly salt and pepper to taste)
- Seaweed sheet with 2 to 3 ounces reduced-fat tuna salad
- 15 olives
- ½ sliced pear and 1½ tablespoons almond butter or another nut butter
- 1 cup sugar snap peas with 3 tablespoons hummus

- 1 cup mixed raw vegetables with 1 tablespoon balsamic vinaigrette
- ½ cup plain low-fat or fat-free plain Greek yogurt mixed with ½ cup blueberries or strawberries and topped with 2 teaspoons chopped nuts and ½ teaspoon organic honey
- ¼ cup guacamole with 1 sliced medium red pepper
- 20 frozen grapes

Exercise

Your exercises for each day are listed below. Now that you are in the third week, it's time to ramp up the exercise a bit to keep your body burning fat. I have added some advanced exercises that you can do at home that don't require any equipment. You can also do them in a gym. All you need is floor space. Please check chapter 13 for instructions on how to do these exercises. You can also find lots of online videos that can show you how to perform the exercises correctly.

| | | | | | | | | | | | | | **DAY 1** | | | | | | | | | | | | | | | |

30 minutes of cardio. Choose a combination of the items below to fulfill your exercise requirement.

Gym Options

- 15 minutes of walking/running on treadmill
- 15 minutes on elliptical machine
- 15 minutes on stationary bicycle
- 15 minutes of swimming laps
- 15 minutes on stair climber
- 15 minutes of spinning
- 15 minutes on rowing machine
- 20 minutes of treadmill intervals

Non-gym Options

- 15 minutes of jogging outside
- 225 jump rope revolutions
- 15 minutes of brisk walking
- 15 minutes of walking up and down a staircase of at least 10 stairs; walking up and down the staircase is considered 1 set (rest between sets as needed)
- 15 minutes of Zumba
- 15 minutes of riding bicycle outside
- 15 minutes of hiking
- 15 minutes of any other high-intensity cardio
- 15 minutes of alternating between running and walking. Run for 1 minute, then walk for 1 minute, then run again and walk again. Repeat the cycle for 15 minutes.

Advanced: Note that doing the exercises as described below will fulfill a 15-minute exercise commitment, even if it doesn't take

15 minutes to complete them. In fact, in most cases, you can finish them in half that time depending on your level of conditioning and how aggressive you are.

- 3 sets of squat jumps (10 consecutive jumps per set)
- 5 sets of mountain climbers (30 seconds of continuous exercise followed by 35 seconds of rest is considered 1 set)
- 3 sets of box jumps (10 consecutive jumps per set)
- 3 sets of tuck jumps (10 consecutive jumps per set)
- 5 sets of ice skaters (35 seconds of exercises followed by 35 seconds of rest is considered 1 set)

DAY 2

30 minutes of cardio. Choose a combination of the items below to fulfill your exercise requirement.

Gym Options

- 15 minutes of walking/running on treadmill
- 15 minutes on elliptical machine
- 15 minutes on stationary bicycle
- 15 minutes of swimming laps
- 15 minutes on stair climber
- 15 minutes of spinning
- 15 minutes on rowing machine
- 20 minutes of treadmill intervals

Non-gym Options

- 15 minutes of jogging outside
- 225 jump rope revolutions
- 15 minutes of brisk walking
- 15 minutes of walking up and down a staircase of at least 10 stairs; walking up and down the staircase is considered 1 set (rest between sets as needed)
- 15 minutes of Zumba
- 15 minutes of riding bicycle outside
- 15 minutes of hiking
- 15 minutes of any other high-intensity cardio
- 15 minutes of alternating between running and walking. Run for 1 minute, then walk for 1 minute, then run again and walk again. Repeat the cycle for 15 minutes.

Advanced: Note that doing the exercises as described below will fulfill a 15-minute exercise commitment, even if it doesn't take

15 minutes to complete them. In fact, in most cases, you can finish them in half that time depending on your level of conditioning and how aggressive you are.

- 3 sets of squat jumps (10 consecutive jumps per set)
- 5 sets of mountain climbers (30 seconds of continuous exercise followed by 35 seconds of rest is considered 1 set)
- 3 sets of box jumps (10 consecutive jumps per set)
- 3 sets of tuck jumps (10 consecutive jumps per set)
- 5 sets of ice skaters (35 seconds of exercises followed by 35 seconds of rest is considered 1 set)

DAY 3

- 10,000 steps throughout the day. Use your wearable device or smartphone to keep track.

| | | | | | | | | | | | | | | **DAY 4** | | | | | | | | | | | | | | | |

40 minutes of cardio broken up into two 20-minute sessions. Choose a combination of the items below to fulfill your exercise requirement.

Gym Options

- 15 minutes of walking/running on treadmill
- 15 minutes on elliptical machine
- 15 minutes on stationary bicycle
- 15 minutes of swimming laps
- 15 minutes on stair climber
- 15 minutes of spinning
- 15 minutes on rowing machine
- 20 minutes of treadmill intervals

Non-gym Options

- 15 minutes of jogging outside
- 225 jump rope revolutions
- 15 minutes of brisk walking
- 15 minutes of walking up and down a staircase of at least 10 stairs; walking up and down the staircase is considered 1 set (rest between sets as needed)
- 15 minutes of Zumba
- 15 minutes of riding bicycle outside
- 15 minutes of hiking
- 15 minutes of any other high-intensity cardio
- 15 minutes of alternating between running and walking. Run for 1 minute, then walk for 1 minute, then run again and walk again. Repeat the cycle for 15 minutes.

Advanced: Note that doing the exercises as described below will fulfill a 15-minute exercise commitment, even if it doesn't take 15 minutes to complete them. In fact, in most cases, you can finish them in half that time depending on your level of conditioning and how aggressive you are.

- 3 sets of squat jumps (10 consecutive jumps per set)
- 5 sets of mountain climbers (30 seconds of continuous exercise followed by 35 seconds of rest is considered 1 set)
- 3 sets of box jumps (10 consecutive jumps per set)
- 3 sets of tuck jumps (10 consecutive jumps per set)
- 5 sets of ice skaters (35 seconds of exercises followed by 35 seconds of rest is considered 1 set)

DAY 5

40 minutes of cardio broken up into two 20-minute sessions. Choose a combination of the items below to fulfill your exercise requirement.

Gym Options
- 15 minutes of walking/running on treadmill
- 15 minutes on elliptical machine
- 15 minutes on stationary bicycle
- 15 minutes of swimming laps
- 15 minutes on stair climber
- 15 minutes of spinning
- 15 minutes on rowing machine
- 20 minutes of treadmill intervals

Non-gym Options
- 15 minutes of jogging outside
- 225 jump rope revolutions
- 15 minutes of brisk walking
- 15 minutes of walking up and down a staircase of at least 10 stairs; walking up and down the staircase is considered 1 set (rest between sets as needed)
- 15 minutes of Zumba
- 15 minutes of riding bicycle outside
- 15 minutes of hiking
- 15 minutes of any other high-intensity cardio
- 15 minutes of alternating between running and walking. Run for 1 minute, then walk for 1 minute, then run again and walk again. Repeat the cycle for 15 minutes.

Advanced: Note that doing the exercises as described below will fulfill a 15-minute exercise commitment, even if it doesn't take 15 minutes to complete them. In fact, in most cases, you can finish them in half that time depending on your level of conditioning and how aggressive you are.

- 3 sets of squat jumps (10 consecutive jumps per set)
- 5 sets of mountain climbers (30 seconds of continuous exercise followed by 35 seconds of rest is considered 1 set)
- 3 sets of box jumps (10 consecutive jumps per set)
- 3 sets of tuck jumps (10 consecutive jumps per set)
- 5 sets of ice skaters (35 seconds of exercises followed by 35 seconds of rest is considered 1 set)

DAY 6

Rest day

DAY 7

You have the choice of two types of workouts. Choose either group A or group B. Each will be effective in its own way.

Group A

15,000 steps throughout the day. Use your wearable device or smartphone to keep track.

20 sets of stairs (up and down is considered 1 set).

Group B

30 minutes of cardio. Choose a combination of the items below.

Gym Options

- 15 minutes of walking/running on treadmill
- 15 minutes on elliptical machine
- 15 minutes on stationary bicycle
- 15 minutes of swimming laps
- 15 minutes on stair climber
- 15 minutes of spinning
- 15 minutes on rowing machine
- 20 minutes of treadmill intervals

Non-gym Options

- 15 minutes of jogging outside
- 225 jump rope revolutions
- 15 minutes of brisk walking
- 15 minutes of walking up and down a staircase of at least 10 stairs; walking up and down the staircase is considered 1 set (rest between sets as needed)
- 15 minutes of Zumba
- 15 minutes of riding bicycle outside
- 15 minutes of hiking

- 15 minutes of any other high-intensity cardio
- 15 minutes of alternating between running and walking. Run for 1 minute, then walk for 1 minute, then run again and walk again. Repeat the cycle for 15 minutes.

Advanced: Note that doing the exercises as described below will fulfill a 15-minute exercise commitment, even if it doesn't take 15 minutes to complete them. In fact, in most cases, you can finish them in half that time depending on your level of conditioning and how aggressive you are.

- 3 sets of squat jumps (10 consecutive jumps per set)
- 5 sets of mountain climbers (30 seconds of continuous exercise followed by 35 seconds of rest is considered 1 set)
- 3 sets of box jumps (10 consecutive jumps per set)
- 3 sets of tuck jumps (10 consecutive jumps per set)
- 5 sets of ice skaters (35 seconds of exercises followed by 35 seconds of rest is considered 1 set)

6

Week 4:
Alternation

THIS IS THE FINAL WEEK OF PART I AND THE LAST WEEK BE-
fore we take a break or intermission. It's important to go into
the break with as much momentum as possible, so that when we re-
emerge for part III, we still are facing forward in the journey to lose
weight and get healthier. This week is all about mixing things up.
We will be alternating between days that are heavily plant-based
and those that are not. If you're a big meat eater, this week might
be a little challenging for you, but it will not be insurmountable. Do
your best to follow the plan as closely as possible. You are still following the 14:10 IF schedule. If you found this too rigorous, then
you can go back to the 12:12, but try your best to do the 14-hour
fasting window.

Guidelines

- You DO NOT have to eat all of the food that's listed. Eat
  enough to satiate. Eat slowly and mindfully enough that
  you can not only taste and enjoy your meals and snacks,
  but notice your body's cues that you are full. Don't eat
  until you're so full that you "can't eat another bite."

- Do your best to fulfill the exercise requirements for the day. You can always break up the exercise into two sessions. What is key is that when you are exercising, you are truly exercising and not just going through the motions. Don't include your breaks in the exercise time.

- These are the beverages allowed during your feeding window. You don't have to drink all of these, but what's listed is the daily maximum. You can have fresh juice (1 cup per day), 2 cups herbal tea (unsweetened), unlimited plain water (still or fizzy), or water with freshly squeezed citrus like lemon or lime.

- You can have some or all of the following: 1 cup freshly squeezed lemonade per day, 2 cups 1% or 2% milk (soy, low-fat, skim, reduced-fat, coconut); 2 cups coffee per day (each coffee must be 50 calories or less).

- If a sandwich calls for cheese, note that it should be 1 slice of cheese of your choice and the size should be approximately 3½ inches square, which is the typical size of packaged cheese.

- NO white bread (100% whole-grain or 100% whole-wheat bread allowed) or products made with white flour.

- NO white pasta (except in the case of chicken noodle soup).

- NO soda (regular or diet).

- NO donuts, cake, brownies, pastries, muffins.

- NO creamy salad dressings.

- NO alcohol.

- NO white potatoes.

- NO frying.

| | | | | | | | | | | | | | | **DAY 1** | | | | | | | | | | | | | | |

Meal 1

- 1 piece of fruit. This can be 1 banana, 1 apple, 1 pear, etc. It can also be ½ cup raspberries, blueberries, blackberries, or strawberries.
- You can have 1 cup fresh juice as well as 1 cup coffee that is less than 50 calories.

Choose one of the following:

- 1 bowl of oatmeal (1½ cups cooked) with 1% or 2% milk, and fresh fruit optional
- 2 egg whites or 1 egg-white omelet with diced veggies and ¼ cup of cheese (made with 2 egg whites max)
- 1 small bowl of sugar-free cereal with fat-free, skim, or 1% or 2% milk
- Herbed Egg-White Wraps (see recipe, page 257)

Snack 1

- Any item 100 calories or less

Meal 2

Choose one of the following:

- Large green salad (all or any of the following: lettuce, 5 olives, 3 tablespoons shredded cheese, 5 cherry tomatoes, 2 tablespoons nuts, sliced cucumbers) with 2 tablespoons low-fat or fat-free vinaigrette-type dressing and 3 ounces sliced chicken or ½ cup beans if desired; no bacon bits and no croutons
- 5-ounce turkey or beef burger on 100% whole-grain bun with one slice of tomato, lettuce, and 1 slice of cheese 3½ inches square

- Tomato and peach salad: In a bowl, combine half of a thinly sliced small red onion, 1 teaspoon red wine vinegar, and a pinch of salt. Slice 1 tomato and 1 peach and arrange on a plate. Drizzle onion mixture over tomato and peach slices. Add ¼ cup crumbled feta if desired.

Snack 2
- Any item 100 calories or less

Meal 3
Choose one of the following:
- 6-ounce piece of grilled or baked chicken or fish with 2 servings of veggies
- 4 servings of vegetables with 1 cup brown rice
- 6-ounce turkey or veggie burger on 100% whole-grain bun with lettuce, 1 slice of cheese 3½ inches square, tomato, and a small green salad
- Honey Glazed Chicken (see recipe, page 278)

Snack 3
- Any item 100 calories or less

Exercise
30 minutes. Choose a combination of the items below to fulfill your exercise requirement.

Gym Options
- 15 minutes of walking/running on treadmill
- 15 minutes on elliptical machine
- 15 minutes on stationary bicycle
- 15 minutes of swimming laps
- 15 minutes on stair climber
- 15 minutes of spinning

- 15 minutes of rowing machine
- 20 minutes of treadmill intervals

Non-gym Options
- 15 minutes of jogging outside
- 225 jump rope revolutions
- 15 minutes of brisk walking
- 15 minutes of walking up and down a staircase of at least 10 stairs; walking up and down the staircase is considered 1 set (rest between sets as needed)
- 15 minutes of Zumba
- 15 minutes of riding bicycle outside
- 15 minutes of hiking
- 15 minutes of any other high-intensity cardio
- 15 minutes of alternating between running and walking. Run for 1 minute, then walk for 1 minute, then run again and walk again. Repeat the cycle for 15 minutes.
- 10 sets of jog punches (45 seconds of active exercise followed by 30 seconds of rest is considered 1 set)

Advanced: Note that doing the exercises as described below will fulfill a 15-minute exercise commitment, even if it doesn't take 15 minutes to complete them. In fact, in most cases, you can finish them in half that time depending on your level of conditioning and how aggressive you are.

- 3 sets of squat jumps (10 consecutive jumps per set)
- 5 sets of mountain climbers (30 seconds of continuous exercise followed by 35 seconds of rest is considered 1 set)
- 3 sets of box jumps (10 consecutive jumps per set)

- 3 sets of tuck jumps (10 consecutive jumps per set)
- 5 sets of ice skaters (35 seconds of exercises followed by 35 seconds of rest is considered 1 set)
- 3 sets of jumping lunges (10 consecutive jumps per set)

| | | | | | | | DAY 2 (Plant-Based) | | | | | | | |

You will be eating four smaller meals today rather than the typical three meals and three snacks. Instead of three snacks, you will have two snacks that you can eat whenever you want throughout the day, as long as you eat them within your feeding window.

Meal 1
Choose one of the following:
- 12-ounce fruit smoothie (300 calories or less)
- 12-ounce protein shake (300 calories or less)
- 8-ounce yogurt parfait (300 calories or less)

Meal 2
Choose one of the following:
- 1½ cups soup (no potato or cream soup like clam chowder). Try the Easy Tomato Soup (see recipe, page 262).
- 4 servings of veggies (cooked or raw)
- Large green salad (all or any of the following: lettuce, 5 olives, 3 tablespoons shredded cheese, 5 cherry tomatoes, 2 tablespoons nuts, sliced cucumbers) with 2 tablespoons low-fat or fat-free vinaigrette-type dressing and 3 ounces sliced chicken or ½ cup beans if desired; no bacon bits and no croutons
- Creamy avocado sandwich: Spread 2 tablespoons low-fat cream cheese over 2 slices of 100% whole-grain or 100% whole-wheat bread, then cut half a ripe avocado into slices and spread over the bread.

Meal 3
Choose one of the following:
- 1½ cups whole-wheat or whole-grain pasta in a marinara sauce with vegetables (squash, broccoli, tomatoes, etc.)

- Large green salad (all or any of the following: lettuce, 5 olives, 3 tablespoons shredded cheese, 5 cherry tomatoes, 2 tablespoons nuts, sliced cucumbers) with 2 tablespoons low-fat or fat-free vinaigrette-type dressing and 3 ounces sliced chicken or ½ cup beans if desired; no bacon bits or croutons
- Roasted Cauliflower (see recipe, page 279) and Moroccan Sweet Potatoes (see recipe, page 280)

Meal 4

Choose one of the following:
- 1½ cups non-creamy soup
- 3 servings of grilled or steamed vegetables and ½ cup brown rice

Choose two snacks from the following list:

- 1 piece of fruit
- 20 raw almonds
- 15 cashews
- 25 dry-roasted peanuts
- 2 tablespoons sunflower or pumpkin seeds
- 1 medium banana
- 2 stalks celery and 4 tablespoons hummus
- 8 baby carrot sticks (or 20 cucumber slices) and 4 tablespoons hummus
- 1 small baked sweet potato
- 2 cups air-popped popcorn with a small amount of salt
- 1 fat-free chocolate or vanilla pudding
- 1½ cups sugar snap peas

- 15 olives
- 1 cup mixed raw vegetables with 1 tablespoon balsamic vinaigrette

Exercise
- 12,000 steps throughout the day. Use your wearable device or smartphone to keep track.

DAY 3

Meal 1
Choose one of the following:
- 1 cup low-fat plain Greek yogurt with fresh fruit
- 12-ounce fresh fruit smoothie (300 calories or less)
- 2 egg whites or 1 egg-white omelet with diced veggies (made with 2 egg whites max)
- 1 small bowl of sugar-free cereal with fat-free, skim, or 1% or 2% milk or ½ cup fresh juice *not* from concentrate (grapefruit, apple, orange juice, tomato, carrot, etc.)

Snack
- Any item 100 calories or less

Meal 2
Choose one of the following:
- Burrito bowl (2 cups brown rice, beans of your choice, tomato, avocado, onion, shredded lettuce)
- Egg salad spread over 1 slice of toasted or untoasted 100% whole-grain or 100% whole-wheat bread (for the egg salad, use 2 whole eggs, low-fat mayo, dill, mustard, chives, salt and pepper)
- Greek Energy Bowl (see recipe, page 260)

Snack
- Any item 100 calories or less

Meal 3
Choose one of the following:
- 1½ cups soup (lentil, black bean, white bean, tomato, squash, vegetable, or cucumber)
- 2 small roasted vegetable and black bean tacos (5-inch diameter)

- Large green salad (all or any of the following: lettuce, 5 olives, 3 tablespoons shredded cheese, 5 cherry tomatoes, 2 tablespoons nuts, sliced cucumbers) with 2 tablespoons vinaigrette-type dressing and 3 ounces sliced chicken or ½ cup beans if desired
- Steak salad (6 ounces thinly sliced steak over a bed of 2 cups arugula, plum tomato cut into wedges, 1 sliced scallion, ⅓ cup sliced pineapple, and 1 tablespoon fresh lime juice)

Snack
- Any item 100 calories or less

Exercise
Rest day

| | | | | | | | DAY 4 (Plant-Based) | | | | | | | |

You will be eating four smaller meals today rather than the typical three meals and three snacks. Instead of three snacks, you will have one snack that you can eat whenever you want during the day, as long as you eat it within your feeding window.

Meal 1
Choose one of the following:
- 12-ounce fruit smoothie (300 calories or less; no sugar added)
- 12-ounce protein shake for breakfast (300 calories or less; no sugar added). Try the Blustery Banana Shake (see recipe, page 289).
- 1 cup oatmeal with optional 1% or 2% milk, fruit, and 1 teaspoon brown sugar
- Cream of Wheat or farina with optional 1% or 2% milk, fruit, and 1 teaspoon brown sugar
- 1 cup grits with optional 1% or 2% milk, fruit, and 1 teaspoon brown sugar

Meal 2
Choose one of the following:
- 1 cup soup (NO cream) with a small green garden salad. Try the Vigorous Vegetable Soup (see page 266).
- 3 servings of veggies (cooked or raw) with ½ cup brown rice
- Black bean bowl (1 cup cooked brown rice; ½ cup black beans; ½ sliced small avocado; and 3 tablespoons shredded cheese, melted or unmelted)
- Spinach salad (3 cups baby spinach, ⅓ cup mushrooms, 5 halved cherry tomatoes, 2 tablespoons chopped red onion, ¼ cup pecan or walnut halves, 1 minced small clove garlic,

and ¼ cup dried cranberries) with 2 tablespoons low-fat or fat-free vinaigrette dressing

Meal 3

Choose one of the following:

- Large green salad (all or any: lettuce, 5 olives, 3 tablespoons shredded cheese, 5 cherry tomatoes, 2 tablespoons nuts, sliced cucumbers) with 2 tablespoons low-fat or fat-free vinaigrette-type dressing and 3 ounces sliced chicken or ½ cup beans if desired; no bacon bits and no croutons
- 1 veggie burger on 100% whole-grain bun with a slice of tomato and a slice of cheese 3½ inches square
- Knockout Brussels Sprouts and brown rice (see recipe, page 282)

Meal 4

Choose one of the following:

- 1 cup soup (NO cream)
- 3 servings of vegetables (cooked or raw) and 1 cup brown rice
- 1 cup cooked whole-wheat pasta with your choice of 2 or 3 veggies and a marinara or lemon white wine sauce

Choose 1 snack from the following list:

- 1 piece of fruit
- 20 raw almonds
- 15 cashews
- 25 dry-roasted peanuts
- 2 tablespoons sunflower or pumpkin seeds
- 1 medium banana and 1 tablespoon cottage cheese
- 2 stalks celery and 4 tablespoons hummus
- 8 baby carrot sticks (or 20 cucumber slices) and 4 tablespoons hummus

- 1 small baked sweet potato
- 2 cups air-popped popcorn with a small amount of salt
- 1 fat-free chocolate or vanilla pudding
- 1½ cups sugar snap peas or edamame
- 15 olives
- 1 cup mixed raw vegetables with 1 tablespoon balsamic vinaigrette

Exercise
- 14,000 steps throughout the day. Use your wearable device or smartphone to keep track.

| | | | | | | | | | | | | | | **DAY 5** | | | | | | | | | | | | | | |

Meal 1
Choose one of the following:
- 1 grilled cheese sandwich (2 slices of cheese 3½ inches square) on 100% whole-grain or 100% whole-wheat bread
- 1 cup low-fat or fat-free plain Greek yogurt with 2 tablespoons granola or muesli and ¼ cup berries

Snack
- Any item 100 calories or less

Meal 2
Choose one of the following:
- Black bean wrap with avocados, diced tomatoes, lettuce, and brown rice on whole-grain tortilla
- Grilled chicken sliders (5-ounce grilled chicken breast sliced on a toasted 100% whole-wheat bun topped with 4 cucumber slices, a slice of tomato, sliced scallions, and 2 tablespoons Thousand Island dressing or dressing of your choice)
- Large green salad (all or any of the following: lettuce, 5 olives, 3 tablespoons shredded cheese, 5 cherry tomatoes, 2 tablespoons nuts, sliced cucumbers) with 2 tablespoons vinaigrette-type dressing and 3 ounces sliced chicken or ½ cup beans if desired

Snack
- Any item 100 calories or less

Meal 3
Choose one of the following:
- 1 serving each of 4 different steamed or raw veggies with ½ cup brown rice

- 1½ cups whole-grain spaghetti with optional diced zucchini, squash, peppers, tomatoes, and/or broccoli in a marinara or lemon-wine sauce
- Grilled chicken salad (lettuce, cucumbers, cherry tomatoes, ½ sliced avocado, 2 tablespoons feta cheese, topped with 5 ounces sliced grilled chicken breast)

Snack:
- Any item 100 calories or less

Exercise
30 minutes of cardio. Choose a combination of the items below to fulfill your exercise requirement.

Gym Options
- 15 minutes of walking/running on treadmill
- 15 minutes on elliptical machine
- 15 minutes on stationary bicycle
- 15 minutes of swimming laps
- 15 minutes on stair climber
- 15 minutes of spinning
- 15 minutes on rowing machine
- 20 minutes of treadmill intervals

Non-gym Options
- 15 minutes of jogging outside
- 225 jump rope revolutions
- 15 minutes of brisk walking
- 15 minutes of walking up and down a staircase of at least 10 stairs; walking up and down the staircase is considered 1 set (rest between sets as needed)
- 15 minutes of Zumba
- 15 minutes of riding bicycle outside

- 15 minutes of hiking
- 15 minutes of any other high-intensity cardio
- 15 minutes of alternating between running and walking. Run for 1 minute, then walk for 1 minute, then run again and walk again. Repeat the cycle for 15 minutes.
- 10 sets of jog punches (45 seconds of active exercise followed by 30 seconds of rest is considered 1 set)

Advanced

Doing the exercises as described will fulfill a 15-minute exercise commitment, even if it doesn't take 15 minutes to complete them. In fact, in most cases, you can finish them in half that time depending on your level of conditioning and how aggressive you are.

- 3 sets of squat jumps (10 consecutive jumps per set)
- 5 sets of mountain climbers (30 seconds of continuous exercise followed by 35 seconds of rest is considered 1 set)
- 3 sets of box jumps (10 consecutive jumps per set)
- 3 sets of tuck jumps (10 consecutive jumps per set)
- 5 sets of ice skaters (35 seconds of exercises followed by 35 seconds of rest is considered 1 set)
- 3 sets of jumping lunges (10 consecutive jumps per set)

| | | | | | | | DAY 6 (Plant-Based) | | | | | | | |

You will be eating four smaller meals today rather than the typical three meals and three snacks. Instead of three snacks, you will have one snack that you can eat whenever you want throughout the day, as long as you eat them within your feeding window.

Meal 1

Choose one of the following:

- 12-ounce fruit smoothie (300 calories or less). Try the Sweet Kale-acious Smoothie (see recipe, page 286).
- 12-ounce protein shake (300 calories or less)
- 1 slice of avocado toast: In a medium bowl, add avocado, ½ teaspoon fresh lemon juice, and salt and pepper to taste, then mash and mix and spread on toasted 100% whole-grain or 100% whole-wheat bread.

Meal 2

Choose one of the following:

- 1½ cups soup. Try the Silky Butternut Squash and Apple Soup (see recipe, page 265).
- 3 servings of veggies (cooked or raw) with ½ cup brown rice
- Veggie wrap with whole-grain or whole-wheat tortilla, vegetables of your choice, and optional slice of cheese 3½ inches square

Meal 3

Choose one of the following:

- Large green salad (all or any: lettuce, 5 olives, 3 tablespoons shredded cheese, 5 cherry tomatoes, 2 tablespoons nuts, sliced cucumbers) with 2 tablespoons low-fat or fat-free vinaigrette-type dressing and 3 ounces sliced chicken or ½ cup beans if desired; no bacon bits and no croutons

- 1½ cups soup (NO cream)
- 1½ cups Victorious Vegan Chili (see recipe, page 261)

Meal 4

Choose one of the following:

- 1½ cups soup
- 4 servings of vegetables, cooked or raw, with ½ cup brown rice
- 1 vegetarian taco in a whole-grain tortilla

Choose 1 snack from the following list:

- 1 piece of fruit
- 20 raw almonds
- 15 cashews
- 25 dry-roasted peanuts
- 2 tablespoons sunflower or pumpkin seeds
- 1 medium banana and 1 tablespoon cottage cheese
- 2 stalks celery and 4 tablespoons hummus
- 8 baby carrot sticks (or 20 cucumber slices) and 4 tablespoons hummus
- 1 small baked sweet potato
- 2 cups air-popped popcorn with a small amount of salt
- 1 fat-free chocolate or vanilla pudding
- 1½ cups sugar snap peas or edamame
- 15 olives
- 1 cup mixed raw vegetables with 1 tablespoon balsamic vinaigrette
- Chocolate-Covered Banana Coins (see recipe, page 284)

Exercise

- 10,000 steps throughout the day. Use your wearable device or smartphone to keep track.

- 15 sets of stairs (up and down is considered 1 set).

DAY 7

Meal 1

Choose one of the following:

- 1 cup oatmeal with optional 1% or 2% milk, fruit, and 1 teaspoon brown sugar
- 1 cup Cream of Wheat or farina with optional 1% or 2% milk, fruit, and 1 teaspoon brown sugar
- 1 cup grits with optional 1% or 2% milk, fruit, and 1 teaspoon brown sugar
- Herbed Egg-White Wraps (see recipe, page 257)

Snack 1

Choose one of the following:

- Raw trail mix (1 cup raw nuts, sunflower or pumpkin seeds, and dried fruit)
- 4 dates stuffed with almonds (take out the pits and replace with a few almonds)
- ½ cup raisins, raw walnuts, and a pinch of sea salt (mix together)
- 2 tomato slices and fresh basil drizzled with olive oil
- 1 medium cucumber, sliced, sprinkled with a pinch of sea salt and fat-free vinaigrette dressing
- 1 cup unsweetened applesauce
- 10 cherries mixed with a handful of nuts (cashews, almonds, or walnuts)
- 8 baby carrots with 2 tablespoons hummus
- Ants on a log (2 celery sticks dabbed with 1 tablespoon raw nut butter and 1 tablespoon organic raisins)
- 1 piece of medium-size fruit
- Small beet or carrot salad

- 1 cup beet or carrot juice
- Chocolate-Covered Banana Coins (see recipe, page 284)

Meal 2

Choose one of the following:
- 1 fruit smoothie (300 calories or less; no sugar added)
- 1 protein shake (300 calories or less; no sugar added)
- 1½ cups soup (no potatoes, no cream). Good choices are chicken noodle, vegetable, lentil, chickpea, split pea, black bean, tomato bisque, etc. Be careful of sodium content! Try for low sodium: 140 mg or less per serving.

Snack 2

Choose one of the following:
- Raw trail mix (½ cup raw nuts, sunflower or pumpkin seeds, and dried fruit)
- 1 date stuffed with almonds (take out the pit and replace with a few almonds)
- ½ cup raisins, raw walnuts, and a pinch of sea salt (mix together)
- 3 tomato slices and fresh basil drizzled with olive oil
- ½ cucumber, sliced, sprinkled with a pinch of sea salt and fat-free vinaigrette dressing
- 1 cup unsweetened applesauce
- 10 cherries mixed with a handful of nuts (cashews, almonds, or walnuts)
- 8 baby carrots with 2 tablespoons hummus
- Ants on a log (2 celery sticks dabbled with 1 tablespoon raw nut butter and 1 tablespoon organic raisins)
- 1 piece of medium-size fruit
- Small beet or carrot salad

- 1 cup beet or carrot juice
- Chocolate-Covered Banana Coins (see recipe, page 284)

Meal 3

Choose one of the following:
- 6-ounce piece of chicken (no skin, no frying) with 2 servings of vegetables
- 6-ounce piece of fish with 2 servings of vegetables
- 6-ounce piece of turkey with 2 servings of vegetables
- 4 servings of vegetables
- Cheesy Whole-Wheat Pasta (1 cup cooked whole-wheat fusilli pasta topped with 1 cup chopped broccoli florets and 3 tablespoons shredded organic Parmesan, with salt and pepper to taste)

Snack 3

Choose one of the following:
- Raw trail mix (½ cup raw nuts, sunflower or pumpkin seeds, and dried fruit)
- 2 dates stuffed with almonds (take out the pits and replace with a few almonds)
- ½ cup raisins, raw walnuts, and a pinch of sea salt (mix together)
- 3 tomato slices and fresh basil drizzled with olive oil
- ½ cucumber, sliced, sprinkled with a pinch of sea salt and fat-free vinaigrette dressing
- 1 cup unsweetened applesauce
- 10 cherries mixed with a handful of nuts (cashews, almonds, or walnuts)
- 8 baby carrots with 2 tablespoons hummus
- Ants on a log (2 celery sticks dabbed with 1 tablespoon raw nut butter and 1 tablespoon organic raisins)

- 1 piece of medium-size fruit
- Small beet or carrot salad
- 1 cup beet or carrot juice
- Chocolate-Covered Banana Coins (see recipe, page 284)

Exercise

30 minutes of cardio as one session or broken up into two. Choose a combination of the items below to fulfill your exercise requirement.

Gym Options

- 15 minutes of walking/running on treadmill
- 15 minutes on elliptical machine
- 15 minutes on stationary bicycle
- 15 minutes of swimming laps
- 15 minutes on stair climber
- 15 minutes of spinning
- 15 minutes on rowing machine
- 20 minutes of treadmill intervals

Non-gym Options

- 15 minutes of jogging outside
- 225 jump rope revolutions
- 15 minutes of brisk walking
- 15 minutes of walking up and down a staircase of at least 10 stairs; walking up and down the staircase is considered 1 set (rest between sets as needed)
- 15 minutes of Zumba
- 15 minutes of riding bicycle outside
- 15 minutes of hiking
- 15 minutes of any other high-intensity cardio
- 15 minutes of alternating between running and walking.

Run for 1 minute, then walk for 1 minute, then run again and walk again. Repeat the cycle for 15 minutes.

- 10 sets of jog punches (45 seconds of active exercise followed by 30 seconds of rest is considered 1 set)

Advanced: Note that doing the exercises as described below will fulfill a 15-minute exercise commitment, even if it doesn't take 15 minutes to complete them. In fact, in most cases, you can finish them in half that time depending on your level of conditioning and how aggressive you are.

- 3 sets of squat jumps (10 consecutive jumps per set)
- 5 sets of mountain climbers (30 seconds of continuous exercise followed by 35 seconds of rest is considered 1 set)
- 3 sets of box jumps (10 consecutive jumps per set)
- 3 sets of tuck jumps (10 consecutive jumps per set)
- 5 sets of ice skaters (35 seconds of exercises followed by 35 seconds of rest is considered 1 set)
- 3 sets of jumping lunges (10 consecutive jumps per set)

PART II

Intermission

7

Week 5:

The Halfway Point

THIS IS A CRITICAL WEEK OF THE PLAN. YOU HAVE REACHED the halfway point! In some respects, you will be taking a bit of a break. There are still guidelines you need to follow, but they are less restrictive, and you will have more liberal choices for your meals and drinks than you had in part I. This week is meant to give your mind and body a chance to reset, but that's not to be confused with reverse. We are not going backward. We must continue to go forward, so that means it's important that you don't revert to making bad decisions and simply eating whatever you want whenever you want. Remember, there's a reason why you've found yourself needing to follow this plan. If what you were doing before was working, then you wouldn't be reading these sentences right now, because you wouldn't be in need of a plan that can help you get back on track. This intermission is only a week, so enjoy it and catch your breath. When you start back up with part III, you'll hit the ground with feet already running. Enjoy this week and have fun.

You can choose whatever IF schedule you want for this week. If you want to go back to the 12:12, by all means feel free to do so. However, just as in the other weeks, once you choose a starting and ending time for your fasting and feeding windows, you must do your best to stick to them for the entire week.

Guidelines

- You will not be prescribed any specific exercise options. Instead, you'll be allowed to choose what you want to do for exercise, as long as your choices meet the time requirement.
- Drink 1 cup of water before every meal, and finish at least 1 cup of water during the meal! Do not take your first bite of food until you have finished the entire first cup of water.
- When you're setting up your fasting and feeding windows, make sure your plan involves not eating your first meal or any solid food until two hours after getting up. Your last solid food of the day must be more than two hours before going to sleep.
- Alcohol is allowed! You are permitted to have four drinks this week. But no more than one drink on any given day. A drink is qualified as a glass of wine, a mixed drink, a bottle of beer or a can of beer.
- Organic honey is allowed.
- Organic 100% stevia is allowed.
- Burritos can be homemade or frozen. If you opt for a frozen burrito, make sure it's low in sodium (300 mg or less per serving).
- If a sandwich calls for cheese, note that it should be 1 slice of cheese of your choice and the size should be approximately 3½ inches square, which is the typical size of packaged cheese.
- NO artificial sweeteners.
- NO frying. The only exception to that directive is that you are allowed to stir-fry veggies in olive oil.

- NO white bread (100% whole-grain or 100% whole-wheat bread allowed).
- NO white pasta (except in the case of chicken noodle soup).
- NO soda.

DAY 1

Meal 1

Choose one of the following:

- 12-ounce fruit smoothie or protein shake
- 2 scrambled eggs with diced veggies, 3 tablespoons shredded cheese (or 1 slice of cheese 3½ inches square) and 1 piece of fruit
- 1 cup steel-cut oats
- 2 pancakes (5 inches in diameter) with 2 tablespoons 100% maple syrup and 1 slice of bacon. Try Gramma's Old-Fashioned Pancakes (see recipe, page 256).

Snack

- Any item 150 calories or less

Meal 2

Choose one of the following:

- Large green garden salad (optional: tomatoes, peppers, 1 hard-boiled egg, ¼ cup chunked avocado, sliced cucumbers) with 3 ounces chicken or fish and 3 tablespoons balsamic vinaigrette
- 1½ cups soup (lentil, black bean, white bean, tomato, or cucumber)
- Turkey or chicken club sandwich on 100% whole-grain or 100% whole-wheat bread with lettuce, tomato, cheese, and choice of 2 tablespoons mustard or 1 tablespoon mayonnaise

Snack

- Any item 150 calories or less

Meal 3

Choose one of the following:

- 1½ cups whole-grain spaghetti with optional diced zucchini, squash, peppers, tomatoes, and/or broccoli in a marinara or lemon-wine sauce
- 4 servings of vegetables with 1 cup brown rice
- Grilled or baked pork chop (½- to 1-inch thick) (see recipe, page 273) with 2 servings of vegetables

Snack

- Any item 150 calories or less

Exercise

30 minutes of cardio.

| | | | | | | | | | | | | | | | **DAY 2** | | | | | | | | | | | | | | | |

Meal 1

Choose one of the following:

- 1 grilled cheese sandwich (2 slices of cheese 3½ inches square) on 100% whole-grain or 100% whole-wheat bread
- 1 cup low-fat or fat-free plain Greek yogurt with ⅓ cup granola or muesli and ¼ cup berries
- 2 scrambled eggs with diced veggies and an optional slice of bacon or slice of 100% whole-grain or 100% whole-wheat toast with butter

Snack

- Any item 150 calories or less

Meal 2

Choose one of the following:

- Black bean wrap with avocados, diced tomatoes, lettuce, and brown rice on whole-grain tortilla
- Large green garden salad (optional: grapefruit, nuts, peppers, tomatoes, sunflower seeds)
- 2 slices of small pizza with your choice of single topping (size is 3 inches wide at the crust and 6 inches long)
- Victorious Vegan Chili (see recipe, page 261)

Snack

- Any item 150 calories or less

Meal 3

Choose one of the following:

- 6-ounce piece of grilled chicken or fish with ¾ cup brown rice and 1 serving of a green vegetable
- 1 serving each of 4 different steamed or raw veggies

- 1½ cups whole-grain spaghetti with optional diced zucchini, squash, peppers, tomatoes, and/or broccoli in a marinara or lemon-wine sauce

Snack
- Any item 150 calories or less

Exercise
- 30 minutes of cardio.

DAY 3

Meal 1

Choose one of the following:

- 1 cup low-fat or fat-free plain Greek yogurt with ⅓ cup muesli and ¼ cup berries
- 1 slice of avocado toast on 100% whole-grain or 100% whole-wheat bread
- 1 cup oatmeal
- 1 cup Cream of Wheat or farina
- 1 cup grits with optional ½ teaspoon butter, 1% or 2% milk, fruit, and ½ teaspoon brown sugar
- 1½ cups cold cereal (7 grams or less sugar) with 1 serving of fruit

Snack

- Any item 150 calories or less

Meal 2

Choose one of the following:

- 1 hummus wrap (hummus, large leaf lettuce, sliced cucumbers, and dill in a whole-grain flour wrap)
- 1 green salad (2 cups greens with 1 cup mixed grapefruit, nuts, peppers, tomatoes, sunflower seeds, orange wedges, and/or cucumbers)
- 6-ounce turkey or beef burger on 100% whole-wheat or 100% whole-grain bun with cheese, tomato, and lettuce and a small green garden salad with 2 tablespoons low-fat or fat-free vinaigrette-type dressing
- Cheesy Chicken Quesadilla (see recipe, page 277)

Snack

- Any item 150 calories or less

Meal 3

Choose one of the following:

- Vegetable stir-fry in olive oil with broccoli, brown rice, peppers, carrots, soy sauce, mushrooms, organic honey
- 1½ cups whole-grain spaghetti with optional diced zucchini, squash, peppers, tomatoes, and/or broccoli in a marinara or lemon-wine sauce
- 6-ounce piece of grilled or baked fish with 2 servings of vegetables

Snack

- Any item 150 calories or less

Exercise

Rest day

DAY 4

Meal 1

Choose one of the following:

- 1 cup low-fat plain Greek yogurt with fresh fruit
- 12-ounce fuit smoothie (300 calories or less; no sugar added). Try Sky Man's Purple Smoothie (see recipe, page 290).
- 2-egg omelet with diced veggies and 3 tablespoons shredded cheese or 1 slice of cheese 3½ inches square

Snack

- Any item 150 calories or less

Meal 2

Choose one of the following:

- Burrito bowl (2 cups brown rice, beans of your choice, tomato, avocado, onion, shredded lettuce)
- Egg salad spread over 1 slice of toasted or untoasted 100% whole-grain or 100% whole-wheat bread (for the egg salad, use 2 whole eggs, low-fat mayo, dill, mustard, chives, salt and pepper)
- 6-ounce turkey or beef burger on 100% whole-grain bun with lettuce, cheese, tomato, and a small green garden salad
- Large green salad (all or any of the following: lettuce, 5 olives, 3 tablespoons shredded cheese, 5 cherry tomatoes, 2 tablespoons nuts, sliced cucumbers) with 2 tablespoons low-fat or fat-free vinaigrette-type dressing and 3 ounces sliced chicken or ½ cup beans if desired; no bacon bits and no croutons

Snack

- Any item 150 calories or less

Meal 3

Choose one of the following:

- 1½ cups soup (lentil, black bean, white bean, tomato, squash, vegetable, or cucumber)
- 2 small roasted vegetable and black bean tacos (6-inch diameter)
- 6-ounce piece of grilled or baked fish or chicken with 2 servings of veggies
- Chickpea Pasta with Pesto (see recipe, page 276)

Snack

- Any item 150 calories or less

Exercise

30 minutes of cardio—break it up into a morning and afternoon/evening session.

| | | | | | | | | | | | | | | | **DAY 5** | | | | | | | | | | | | | | | |

Meal 1

Choose one of the following:

- 12-ounce fresh smoothie or protein shake (300 calories or less; no sugar added)
- 1 cup steel-cut oats with optional sliced apples, walnuts, 1% or 2% milk, and ½ teaspoon brown sugar
- 2 scrambled eggs with diced veggies and an optional slice of bacon or slice of 100% whole-grain or 100% whole-wheat toast with butter

Snack

- Any item 150 calories or less

Meal 2

Choose one of the following:

- 2 cups bean salad (tomato, cucumber, onion, and black or white beans with 2 tablespoons balsamic vinaigrette)
- Lettuce, cheese, tomato sandwich on 100% whole-grain or 100% whole-wheat toast with your choice of spread
- 2 slices of small pizza with your choice of single topping (size is 4 inches wide at the crust and 6 inches long)
- Silky Butternut Squash and Apple Soup (see recipe, page 265)

Snack

- Any item 150 calories or less

Meal 3

Choose one of the following:

- Cauliflower and brown rice stuffed peppers (both halves of a small pepper)

- Portobello mushroom steaks: First marinate in spices and soy sauce or balsamic vinaigrette, then cook with a touch of olive oil and salt and pepper to taste.
- Grilled or baked pork chop (½- to 1-inch thick) (see recipe, page 273) with 2 servings of vegetables

Snack

- Any item 150 calories or less

Exercise

30 minutes of cardio.

|||||||||||||||||| DAY 6 |||||||||||||||||||

Meal 1
Choose one of the following:

- 2-egg omelet with diced veggies and 3 tablespoons shredded cheese or 1 slice of cheese 3½ inches squre

- 12-ounce fruit smoothie or protein shake (350 calories or less; no sugar added). Try the Blustery Banana Shake (see recipe, page 289).

- 1 cup oatmeal with optional 1% or 2% milk, fruit, and ½ teaspoon brown sugar

- 1 cup Cream of Wheat or farina with optional 1% or 2% milk, fruit, and ½ teaspoon brown sugar

- 1 cup grits with optional 1% or 2% milk, fruit, and ½ teaspoon brown sugar

Snack
- Any item 150 calories or less

Meal 2
Choose one of the following:

- 1½ cups cabbage soup

- Veggie and hummus sandwich on 100% whole-grain or 100% whole-wheat bread

- 6-ounce turkey or beef burger on 100% whole-wheat or 100% whole-grain bun with cheese, tomato, and lettuce and a small green garden salad with 2 tablespoons low-fat or fat-free vinaigrette-type dressing

Snack
- Any item 150 calories or less

Meal 3

Choose one of the following:

- Bean, vegetable, cheese enchilada on 6-inch whole-grain flour tortilla
- 1½ cups poke bowl with brown rice, avocado, edamame, cucumber
- 6-ounce piece of fish or chicken with 2 servings of veggies
- Tender Baked Pork Chops (see recipe, page 273)

Snack

- Any item 150 calories or less

Exercise

Rest day

| | | | | | | | | | | | | | **DAY 7** | | | | | | | | | | | | | |

Meal 1
Choose one of the following:
- 1½ cups cold cereal (7 grams or less sugar)
- 2-egg omelet with diced veggies and 3 tablespoons shredded cheese or 1 slice of cheese 3½ inches square
- 2 pancakes (5 inches in diameter) with 2 tablespoons 100% maple syrup and 1 slice of bacon

Snack
- Any item 150 calories or less

Meal 2
Choose one of the following:
- 2 slices of tomato-cheese toast on 100% whole-grain or 100% whole-wheat bread
- Bean burrito with cheese and sour cream in 6-inch whole-grain flour tortilla (use low-sodium black or refried beans)
- 6-ounce turkey or beef burger on 100% whole-grain bun with lettuce, cheese, tomato, and a small green garden salad

Snack
- Any item 150 calories or less

Meal 3
Choose one of the following:
- Vegetable stir-fry in olive oil with broccoli, brown rice, peppers, carrots, soy sauce, mushrooms, organic honey
- 1½ cups non-creamy soup with a small green garden salad
- 2 slices of small pizza with your choice of single topping (size is 4 inches wide at the crust and 6 inches long)
- Beef Burrito Bowl (see recipe, page 268)

Snack

- Any item 150 calories or less

Exercise

30 minutes of cardio—break it up into a morning and afternoon/evening session.

PART III

Acceleration

8

Week 6:
Reload

NOW THAT YOU'VE HAD TIME TO RESET AND TAKE A breather during intermission, it's time to reload your weapons as you attack the second and final part of **FAST BURN**. After being on the plan for five weeks, I hope you've learned some new things about yourself and that you've picked up some positive eating and exercising behaviors and attitudes that will permanently become a part of who you are and how you will conduct your life going forward.

We only have four weeks left, so there's no time to fiddle and diddle. You need to get right back at it and be even more aggressive. You're asking for your body to deliver great results, so you must be willing to put in the appropriate effort to achieve those results. Part III is called **ACCELERATION**, because we are going to tighten and advance your requirements on the plan and push your body to accelerate the process of burning fat and those unwanted pounds. The daily meal plans in this part are written very specifically, so follow them as closely as possible. The weeks are not all the same, so it's imperative that you pay attention to the details. There are going to be some different elements introduced in some of the following weeks that you haven't seen before but should be exciting and beneficial. You will see something called the **Daily Double,** where you get to double your calories that day. There is also something called a **Floating Bonus Snack,** where you get an extra snack that day in the event you need a little extra infusion of calories and nutrients.

For this week specifically, your IF schedule should be 14:10; for those who are choosing a more aggressive approach, you should move up to 16:8. Do as much of your exercise as possible within your fasting window, because one of the important strategies this week is increasing your energy demand while decreasing your energy supply from food. This will continue to drive your body more into your fat stores to break them down to make more energy available. Let's reload and get back in the fight!

Guidelines

- If you don't eat meat, make the substitutions appropriately with fish or vegetables.
- Soups can be consumed with 2 saltine crackers if desired.
- The liquid meals must be eaten with either 1 piece of fruit or 1 serving of vegetables.
- You must consume 1 cup water before eating a meal; you must consume 1 cup water during your meal. You can add lemon or lime to your water, and you can drink fizzy water if you desire.
- If a sandwich calls for cheese, note that it should be 1 slice of cheese of your choice and the size should be approximately 3½ inches square, which is the typical size of packaged cheese.
- You can drink coffee, but only 1 small cup per day. Stay away from all of those fancy coffee preparations that have lots of calories. Your coffee should contain no more than 50 calories.

- Don't eat your first meal until two hours after you are awake.

- Do not eat the last meal within two hours of going to sleep. You can eat a 100-calorie snack before going to bed if desired.

- Be smart in your snack choices. Avoid chips and donuts and candy; you can have them some of the time, but don't eat them often. They must fall within the calorie limit as described in the daily meal plan if you decide to have them, but please note these are not smart snacks or beneficial to your long-term goals. If you must have something like these items, make it only one of your snacks for the day and use healthier options for the other snacks.

- You don't have to eat all of the food on the day's menu if you don't want to, but no skipping meals, no doubling up on meals, and no exceeding the meal guidelines in size and volume.

- Condiments such as ketchup, mayo, and mustard are allowed, but no more than 2 tablespoons at each meal for ketchup and mustard and 1 tablespoon for mayo; 2 to 3 tablespoons low-sodium soy sauce is allowed.

- Spices are unlimited.

- While fresh fruit is always preferred, canned and frozen fruit are allowed. Just make sure they are water-based and there are no added sugars.

- Canned and frozen vegetables are allowed. Please be aware of the sodium content. Try for low sodium: 140 mg or less per serving.

- As far as beverages are concerned, you are allowed as much water as you like per day. Here are some other beverage guidelines: flavored waters are allowed, but keep them under 60 calories; 1 bottle of sports drink allowed per day, but keep it under 60 calories.

- No white bread (100% whole-grain or 100% whole-wheat bread allowed).
- No alcohol.
- No soda.
- No fried food.
- No white pasta (except in the case of chicken noodle soup).

| | | | | | | | | | | | | | | | **DAY 1** | | | | | | | | | | | | | | | | | |

Meal 1

Choose one of the following:

- 1 cup oatmeal with optional 1% or 2% milk, fruit, and ½ teaspoon brown sugar
- 2 egg whites or 1 egg-white omelet with diced veggies (made with 2 egg whites)
- 1 small bowl of sugar-free cereal with fat-free, skim, or 1% or 2% milk with 1 serving of fruit
- 8-ounce yogurt parfait with ¼ cup berries and ⅓ cup granola

Snack 1

- Any item 100 calories or less

Meal 2

Choose one of the following:

- Large green garden salad with 3 ounces chicken or fish if desired. Only 2 tablespoons fat-free or low-fat vinaigrette-type dressing, no bacon bits, no croutons. Keep it clean.
- 1½ cups soup (lentil, black bean, white bean, tomato, or cucumber) with a small green salad
- Roasted Cauliflower (see recipe, page 279) with 1 cup brown rice and 1 serving of a green vegetable

Snack 2

- Any item 150 calories or less

Meal 3

Choose one of the following:

- 6-ounce piece of grilled or baked chicken or fish with 2 servings of veggies. Try the Honey Glazed Chicken (see recipe, page 278).

- 1½ cups whole-grain spaghetti with optional diced zucchini, squash, peppers, tomatoes, and/or broccoli in a marinara or lemon-wine sauce
- Portobello mushroom steaks: First marinate in spices and soy sauce or balsamic vinaigrette, then cook with a touch of olive oil and salt and pepper to taste.

Exercise

40 minutes. Break it up into 2 sessions during the day. Choose 2 of the following exercises for a total of 40 minutes.

Gym Options

- 20 minutes of walking/running on treadmill
- 20 minutes on elliptical machine
- 20 minutes on stationary bicycle
- 20 minutes of swimming laps
- 20 minutes on stair climber
- 20 minutes of spinning
- 20 minutes on rowing machine
- 20 minutes of treadmill intervals

Non-gym Options

- 10 sets of butt kicks (35 seconds of exercise followed by 35 seconds of rest is considered 1 set)
- 10 sets of line hops (35 seconds of exercise followed by 35 seconds of rest is considered 1 set)
- 15 minutes of jogging outside
- 225 jump rope revolutions
- 20 minutes of brisk walking
- 20 minutes of walking up and down a staircase of at least 10 stairs; walking up and down the staircase is considered 1 set (rest between sets as needed)

- 20 minutes of Zumba
- 20 minutes of riding bicycle outside
- 20 minutes of hiking
- 20 minutes of any other high-intensity cardio
- 20 minutes of alternating between running and walking. Run for 1 minute, then walk for 1 minute, then run again and walk again. Repeat the cycle for 15 minutes.
- 10 sets of jog punches (45 seconds of active exercise followed by 30 seconds of rest is considered 1 set)

Advanced

Doing the exercises as described will fulfill a 15-minute exercise commitment, even if it doesn't take 15 minutes to complete them. In fact, in most cases, you can finish them in half that time depending on your level of conditioning and how aggressive you are.

- 3 sets of squat jumps (10 consecutive jumps per set)
- 5 sets of mountain climbers (30 seconds of continuous exercise followed by 35 seconds of rest is considered 1 set)
- 3 sets of box jumps (10 consecutive jumps per set)
- 3 sets of tuck jumps (10 consecutive jumps per set)
- 5 sets of ice skaters (35 seconds of exercises followed by 35 seconds of rest is considered 1 set)
- 3 sets of jumping lunges (10 consecutive jumps per set)

|||||||||||||| **DAY 2** ||||||||||||||||

Meal 1

Choose 1 of the following:

- 12-ounce fruit smoothie (300 calories or less; no sugar added)
- 12-ounce veggie smoothie (300 calories or less; no sugar added)
- 12-ounce protein shake (300 calories or less; no sugar added)
- 1 cup steel-cut oats (optional: berries, bananas, cinnamon) with 2 slices of bacon optional

Snack 1

Choose from the following:

- 30 grapes
- 1½ cups sugar snap peas
- 1 cup sliced zucchini, seasoned to taste
- 1 rice cake with 1 tablespoon guacamole
- 17 pecans
- 20 olives
- 1 medium grapefruit sprinkled with ½ teaspoon sugar
- 1 can tuna (canned in water), seasoned to taste
- 1½ cups diced watermelon
- 14 raw almonds
- ½ small cucumber, sliced, with 2 tablespoons hummus
- 8 baby carrots with 2 tablespoons hummus
- 1 celery stalk, cut into sticks, with 2 tablespoons hummus

Meal 2

Choose one of the following:

- 3 servings of vegetables. One of the vegetables must be a dark-green leafy vegetable, such as spinach, kale, lettuce, mustard greens, collard greens, chicory, or Swiss chard. One must also be some type of legume (lentils, peas, chickpeas, soybeans, black beans, white beans, red beans, lima beans, mung beans, pinto beans, navy beans, black-eyed peas, etc.).
- Large green salad (all or any: lettuce, 5 olives, 3 tablespoons shredded cheese, 5 cherry tomatoes, 2 tablespoons nuts, sliced cucumbers) with 2 tablespoons low-fat or fat-free vinaigrette-type dressing and 3 ounces sliced chicken or ½ cup beans if desired; no bacon bits and no croutons
- 1 cup brown rice or quinoa with 1 cup legumes
- Moroccan Sweet Potatoes (see recipe, page 280) with 2 servings of other vegetables

Snack 2

- Any item 150 calories or less

Meal 3

Choose one of the following:

- Large green garden salad with 5 ounces chicken or fish if desired (no croutons, no bacon bits; 2 tablespoons fat-free or low-fat vinaigrette-type dressing)
- 6 ounces steamed shrimp or baked fish topped with 3 tablespoons salsa and served with 1 small baked sweet potato and 1 serving of green veggie of your choice
- Grilled pork chop covered in a mixture of 2 tablespoons Italian salad dressing, 1 tablespoon soy sauce, and ¼ teaspoon pepper over a bed of brown rice with a side of asparagus

- 1 serving of lasagna (with or without meat, 4 by 3 by 1 inch)
- 1 veggie burger (3 inches in diameter, ½-inch thick) with 2 servings of vegetables

Snack 3

Choose one of the following:

- 30 grapes
- 1½ cups sugar snap peas
- 1 cup sliced zucchini, seasoned to taste
- 1 rice cake with 1 tablespoon guacamole
- 17 pecans
- 20 olives
- 1 medium grapefruit sprinkled with ½ teaspoon sugar
- 1 can tuna (canned in water), seasoned to taste
- 1½ cups diced watermelon
- 1 apple
- 1 pear
- 1½ cups air-popped popcorn
- 10 cherries mixed with a handful of nuts (cashews, almonds, or walnuts)
- 8 baby carrots with 2 tablespoons hummus
- Kale chips
- 1½ cups veggie juice (not from concentrate)

Exercise

40 minutes. Choose 2 of the following exercises for a total of 40 minutes.

Gym Options

- 20 minutes of walking/running on treadmill
- 20 minutes on elliptical machine

- 20 minutes on stationary bicycle
- 20 minutes of swimming laps
- 20 minutes on stair climber
- 20 minutes of spinning
- 20p minutes on rowing machine
- 20 minutes of treadmill intervals

Non-gym Options

- 10 sets of butt kicks (35 seconds of exercise followed by 35 seconds of rest is considered 1 set)
- 10 sets of line hops (35 seconds of exercise followed by 35 seconds of rest is considered 1 set)
- 20 minutes of jogging outside
- 225 jump rope revolutions
- 20 minutes of brisk walking
- 20 minutes of walking up and down a staircase of at least 10 stairs; walking up and down the staircase is considered 1 set (rest between sets as needed)
- 20 minutes of Zumba
- 20 minutes of riding bicycle outside
- 20 minutes of hiking
- 20 minutes of any other high-intensity cardio
- 20 minutes of alternating between running and walking. Run for 1 minute, then walk for 1 minute, then run again and walk again. Repeat the cycle for 15 minutes.
- 10 sets of jog punches (45 seconds of active exercise followed by 30 seconds of rest is considered 1 set)

Advanced

Doing the exercises as described below will fulfill a 15-minute exercise commitment, even if it doesn't take 15 minutes to complete them. In fact, in most cases, you can finish them in half that time depending on your level of conditioning and how aggressive you are.

- 3 sets of squat jumps (10 consecutive jumps per set)
- 5 sets of mountain climbers (30 seconds of continuous exercise followed by 35 seconds of rest is considered 1 set)
- 3 sets of box jumps (10 consecutive jumps per set)
- 3 sets of tuck jumps (10 consecutive jumps per set)
- 5 sets of ice skaters (35 seconds of exercises followed by 35 seconds of rest is considered 1 set)
- 3 sets of jumping lunges (10 consecutive jumps per set)

| | | | | | | | | | | | | | | | | | | | **DAY 3** | | | | | | | | | | | | | | | | | |

Meal 1

Choose one of the following. Your portion should be 1 cup cooked.

- 1 small bowl of oatmeal with optional fruit, 1% or 2% milk, and 1 teaspoon brown sugar
- 1 small bowl of Cream of Wheat or farina with optional fruit, 1% or 2% milk, and 1 teaspoon brown sugar
- 1 small bowl of grits with optional fruit, 1% or 2% milk, and 1 teaspoon brown sugar
- 8-ounce yogurt parfait
- 12-ounce protein shake (300 calories or less; no sugar added). Try the Creamy Chocolate Shake (see recipe, page 288).

Snack 1

Choose one of the following:

- 30 grapes
- 1½ cups sugar snap peas
- 1 cup sliced zucchini, seasoned to taste
- 1 rice cake with 1 tablespoon guacamole
- 17 pecans
- 20 olives
- 1 medium grapefruit sprinkled with ½ teaspoon sugar
- 1 can tuna (canned in water), seasoned to taste
- 1½ cups diced watermelon
- Raw trail mix (1 cup raw nuts, sunflower or pumpkin seeds, and dried fruit)
- 4 dates stuffed with almonds (take out the pits and replace with a few almonds)

- ½ cup raisins, raw walnuts, and a pinch of sea salt (mix together)
- 2 tomato slices and fresh basil drizzled with olive oil
- ½ small cucumber, sliced, sprinkled with a pinch of sea salt and fat-free vinaigrette dressing
- 1 cup unsweetened applesauce
- 10 cherries mixed with a handful of nuts (cashews, almonds, or walnuts)
- 8 baby carrots with 2 tablespoons hummus
- Ants on a log (2 celery sticks dabbed with 1 tablespoon raw nut butter and 1 tablespoon organic raisins)
- 1 piece of medium-size fruit
- Small beet or carrot salad
- 1 cup beet or carrot juice

Meal 2

Choose one of the following. Your choice must be 300 calories or less.

- 1½ cups soup (no potatoes, no cream) with 1 serving of veggies. Good choices are chicken noodle, vegetable, lentil, chickpea, split pea, black bean, tomato bisque, etc. Be careful of sodium content. Try for low sodium: 140 mg or less per serving.
- Veggie and hummus sandwich on 100% whole-grain or 100% whole-wheat bread
- Burrito bowl (2 cups brown rice, beans of your choice, tomato, avocado, onion, shredded lettuce)
- Knockout Brussels Sprouts (see recipe, page 282) with 1 cup brown rice

Snack 2

Choose one of the following:

- 30 grapes
- 1½ cups sugar snap peas
- 1 cup sliced zucchini, seasoned to taste
- 1 rice cake with 1 tablespoon guacamole
- 17 pecans
- 20 olives
- 1 medium grapefruit sprinkled with ½ teaspoon sugar
- 1 can tuna (canned in water), seasoned to taste
- 1½ cups diced watermelon
- Raw trail mix (½ cup raw nuts, sunflower or pumpkin seeds, and dried fruit)
- 1 date stuffed with almonds (take out the pit and replace with a few almonds)
- ½ cup raisins, raw walnuts, and a pinch of sea salt (mix together)
- 3 tomato slices and fresh basil drizzled with olive oil
- ½ cucumber, sliced, sprinkled with a pinch of sea salt and fat-free vinaigrette dressing
- 1 cup unsweetened applesauce
- 10 cherries mixed with a handful of nuts (cashews, almonds, or walnuts)
- 8 baby carrots with 2 tablespoons hummus
- Ants on a log (2 celery sticks dabbed with 1 tablespoon raw nut butter and 1 tablespoon organic raisins)
- 1 piece of medium-size fruit
- Small beet or carrot salad
- 1 cup beet or carrot juice

Meal 3

Choose one of the following:

- 6-ounce piece of chicken with 1 serving of vegetables and 1 cup brown rice
- Tomato Pesto Pasta (1 cup cooked whole-wheat penne pasta with 2 tablespoons pesto and 5 halved cherry tomatoes cooked in a skillet in olive oil until soft)
- 6-ounce piece of fish with 1 serving of vegetables and 1 cup brown rice
- 6-ounce piece of turkey with 1 serving of vegetables and 1 cup brown rice
- 4 servings of vegetables and ½ cup brown rice

Snack 3

Choose one of the following:

- 30 grapes
- 1½ cups sugar snap peas
- 1 cup sliced zucchini, seasoned to taste
- 1 rice cake with 1 tablespoon guacamole
- 17 pecans
- 20 olives
- 1 medium grapefruit sprinkled with ½ teaspoon sugar
- 1 can tuna (canned in water), seasoned to taste
- 1½ cups diced watermelon
- Raw trail mix (½ cup raw nuts, sunflower or pumpkin seeds, and dried fruit)
- 2 dates stuffed with almonds (take out the pits and replace with a few almonds)
- ½ cup raisins, raw walnuts, and a pinch of sea salt (mix together)
- 3 tomato slices and fresh basil drizzled with olive oil

- ½ small cucumber, sliced, sprinkled with a pinch of sea salt and fat-free vinaigrette dressing
- 1 cup unsweetened applesauce
- 10 cherries mixed with a handful of nuts (cashews, almonds, or walnuts)
- 8 baby carrots with 2 tablespoons hummus
- Ants on a log (2 celery sticks dabbed with 1 tablespoon raw nut butter and 1 tablespoon organic raisins)
- 1 piece of medium-size fruit
- Small beet or carrot salad
- 1 cup beet or carrot juice

Exercise

- 12,000 steps throughout the day. Use your wearable device or smartphone to keep track.

DAY 4

Meal 1
Choose one of the following:
- 12-ounce protein shake (300 calories or less, no added sugar). Try the Sumptuous Strawberry Shake (see recipe, page 287).
- 12-ounce fruit smoothie (300 calories or less; no added sugar)

Snack
- Any item 150 calories or less

Meal 2
Choose one of the following:
- Large green salad (all or any of the following: lettuce, 5 olives, 3 tablespoons shredded cheese, 5 cherry tomatoes, 2 tablespoons nuts, sliced cucumbers) with 2 tablespoons low-fat or fat-free vinaigrette-type dressing and 3 ounces sliced chicken or ½ cup beans if desired; no bacon bits and no croutons
- Broccoli cheddar quesadilla: Place a 10-inch whole-wheat tortilla in a skillet over medium heat, spread cooked broccoli over the tortilla, top with 3 tablespoons shredded cheddar cheese and fold over. Cook on both sides until cheese melts and tortilla is golden brown.
- 1 cup cooked beans, chickpeas, or lentils (no baked beans) with 1 cup brown rice
- Crunchy Chipper Chickpeas (see recipe, page 283) with 1 cup brown rice

Snack
- Any item 150 calories or less

Meal 3

Choose one of the following:

- 4 servings of vegetables, raw or cooked, with ½ cup brown rice
- 12-ounce protein shake (300 calories or less; no sugar added)
- 1 cup whole-grain pasta in a meatless tomato sauce with 1 serving of veggies mixed into the pasta

Exercise

- 14,000 steps throughout the day. Use your wearable device or smartphone to keep track.
- 15 sets of stairs (up and down at least 10 steps is considered 1 set)

DAY 5

Meal 1

Choose one of the following:

- 12-ounce protein shake (300 calories or less, no added sugar)
- 12-ounce fruit smoothie (300 calories or less; no added sugar)
- 8-ounce yogurt parfait with low-fat plain Greek yogurt, ¼ cup granola or nuts, and ⅓ cup berries
- 2 scrambled eggs with diced veggies and 3 tablespoons shredded cheese (or 1 slice of cheese 3½ inches square)

Snack

- Any item 150 calories or less

Meal 2

Choose one of the following:

- Large green salad (3 cups greens) with 2 tablespoons fat-free or low-fat vinaigrette-type dressing (options: 5 olives, 3 tablespoons shredded cheese, 6 cherry tomatoes, ¼ cup nuts, ½ hard-boiled egg, sliced cucumbers; no bacon, no croutons, no ham)
- Shrimp salad: Cook 4 shrimp in a skillet over medium heat, then add ½ cup corn and ½ cup black beans, salt, and pepper. Cook for 3 to 5 minutes, then serve.
- 1½ cups soup (options: black bean, white bean, tomato, gazpacho, lentil, chickpea, vegetable, squash, pea, chicken noodle); NO creamy or potato soups

Snack

- Any item 150 calories or less

Meal 3

Choose one of the following:

- 4 servings of vegetables, raw or cooked with ½ cup brown rice
- 12-ounce protein shake (300 calories or less; no sugar added)
- Large green salad (3 cups greens) with 2 tablespoons low-fat or fat-free vinaigrette-type dressing (options: 5 olives, 3 tablespoons shredded cheese, 6 cherry tomatoes, ¼ cup nuts, ½ hard-boiled egg, sliced cucumbers; no bacon, no croutons, no ham)
- Supreme Strip Steak (see recipe, page 275)

Exercise

- Walk 14,000 steps throughout the day. Use your wearable device or smartphone to keep track.

| | | | | | | | | | | | | | | **DAY 6** | | | | | | | | | | | | | | | |

Meal 1

Choose one of the following:

- 12-ounce protein shake (300 calories or less, no added sugar)
- 12-ounce fruit smoothie (300 calories or less; no added sugar). Try the Sweet Kale-acious Smoothie (see recipe, page 286).
- 1 fruit plate (½ sliced apple, ½ sliced grapefruit, 3 slices melon)
- 8-ounce yogurt parfait with 2 tablespoons granola and ¼ cup berries

Snack

- Any item 150 calories or less

Meal 2

Choose one of the following:

- 4 servings of cooked or raw vegetables with ½ cup brown rice
- 1½ cups soup (options: black bean, white bean, tomato, gazpacho, lentil, chickpea, vegetable, squash, pea, chicken noodle); NO creamy or potato soups
- Mango Curry Chickpeas (see recipe, page 281) with 1 cup brown rice

Snack

- Any item 150 calories or less

Meal 3

Choose one of the following:

- 4 servings of vegetables, raw or cooked with ½ cup brown rice

- 12-ounce protein shake (350 calories or less; no sugar added)
- Large green salad (all or any: lettuce, 5 olives, 3 tablespoons shredded cheese, 5 cherry tomatoes, 2 tablespoons nuts, sliced cucumbers) with 2 tablespoons low-fat or fat-free vinaigrette-type dressing and 3 ounces sliced chicken or ½ cup beans if desired; no bacon bits and no croutons

Exercise
Rest day

Meal 1

Choose one of the following:

- 12-ounce protein shake (300 calories or less; no added sugar)
- 12-ounce fruit smoothie (300 calories or less; no sugar added)
- Egg-white omelet with diced veggies and a slice of cheese (use 2 to 3 egg whites and 1 slice of cheese 3½ inches square)
- Baked Apple Heaven (see recipe, page 255)

Snack

- Any item 150 calories or less

Meal 2

Choose one of the following:

- Large green salad (all or any of the following: lettuce, 5 olives, 3 tablespoons shredded cheese, 5 cherry tomatoes, 2 tablespoons nuts, sliced cucumbers, ½ hard-boiled egg) with 2 tablespoons low-fat or fat-free vinaigrette-type dressing and 3 ounces sliced chicken or ½ cup beans if desired; no bacon bits and no croutons
- Hummus chicken salad: In a bowl, combine ¾ cup shredded or diced cooked chicken and ⅓ cup hummus of your preferred flavor and spread between 2 pieces of 100% whole-grain or 100% whole-wheat bread.
- 2 slices of small cheese pizza (no larger than 3 inches across the crust and 6 inches long) with 1 serving of vegetables or a small salad

Snack
- Any item 150 calories or less

Meal 3
Choose one of the following:
- 4 servings of vegetables, raw or cooked, with ½ cup brown rice
- 12-ounce protein shake (300 calories or less; no added sugar)
- 1 cup whole-grain pasta in a meatless tomato sauce with 1 serving of veggies mixed into the pasta

Exercise
40 minutes of cardio broken up into 2 sessions. Choose 2 of the following exercises for a total of 40 minutes.

Gym Options
- 15 minutes of walking/running on treadmill
- 15 minutes on elliptical machine
- 15 minutes on stationary bicycle
- 15 minutes of swimming laps
- 15 minutes on stair climber
- 15 minutes of spinning
- 15 minutes on rowing machine
- 20 minutes of treadmill intervals

Non-gym Options
- 10 sets of butt kicks (35 seconds of exercise followed by 35 seconds of rest is considered 1 set)
- 10 sets of line hops (35 seconds of exercise followed by 35 seconds of rest is considered 1 set)
- 15 minutes of jogging outside
- 225 jump rope revolutions

- 15 minutes of brisk walking
- 15 minutes of walking up and down a staircase of at least 10 stairs; walking up and down the staircase is considered 1 set (rest between sets as needed)
- 15 minutes of Zumba
- 15 minutes of riding bicycle outside
- 15 minutes of hiking
- 15 minutes of any other high-intensity cardio
- 15 minutes of alternating between running and walking. Run for 1 minute, then walk for 1 minute, then run again and walk again. Repeat the cycle for 15 minutes.
- 10 sets of jog punches (45 seconds of active exercise followed by 30 seconds of rest is considered 1 set)

Advanced

Doing the exercises as described below will fulfill a 15-minute exercise commitment, even if it doesn't take 15 minutes to complete them. In fact, in most cases, you can finish them in half that time depending on your level of conditioning and how aggressive you are.

- 3 sets of squat jumps (10 consecutive jumps per set)
- 5 sets of mountain climbers (30 seconds of continuous exercise followed by 35 seconds of rest is considered 1 set)
- 3 sets of box jumps (10 consecutive jumps per set)
- 3 sets of tuck jumps (10 consecutive jumps per set)
- 5 sets of ice skaters (35 seconds of exercises followed by 35 seconds of rest is considered 1 set)
- 3 sets of jumping lunges (10 consecutive jumps per set)

9

Week 7:

Jigsaw Week #2

THIS IS A PLANT-BASED WEEK. IT'S NOT TOTALLY VEGETAR-
ian, but it relies predominantly on non-animal products. If
you follow this week as written, you will definitely burn fat and
lose weight. Try to stick to the guidelines and meal options as
much as possible. If you slip a little, don't get upset, just try to do
better. This is similar to the first jigsaw you had in week 3. You decide your daily meal plans based on the options listed below. Try
to choose a variety of foods so that you don't get bored with eating
the same meals. This is important, because lack of diversity in a
meal plan can be an enticement to stray off the plan because you're
not excited by the food choices. Your IF schedule this week should
be 14:10 or 16:8.

These are the kinds of foods and ingredients you should be focusing on:

- Vegetables (including kale, spinach, Swiss chard, collard
  greens, sweet potatoes, asparagus, bell peppers, and
  broccoli)
- Fruits (such as avocado, strawberries, blueberries,
  watermelon, apples, grapes, bananas, grapefruit, and
  oranges)

- Whole grains (such as quinoa, farro, brown rice, whole-wheat bread, and whole-wheat pasta)
- Nuts (such as walnuts, almonds, macadamia nuts, and cashews)
- Seeds (such as flaxseeds, chia seeds, and hemp seeds)
- Beans
- Lentils
- Coffee
- Tea (including green, lavender, chamomile, or ginger)

These are the kinds of foods and ingredients you should be avoiding or reducing to limited quantities:

- Meat and poultry (like chicken, beef, and pork)
- Processed animal meats, such as sausages and hot dogs
- All animal products (including eggs, dairy, and meat if you're following a vegan diet)
- Refined grains (such as "white" foods, like white pasta, rice, and bread)
- Sweets (like cookies, brownies, and cake)
- Sweetened beverages (such as soda and fruit juice)
- Potatoes and French fries
- Honey (if you're strict vegan)
- Hydrogenated oils
- High-fructose corn syrup
- MSG (monosodium glutamate)
- Sucralose and aspartame
- Artificial flavors
- Artificial colors (may just be listed as "blue," for example)

- Preservatives such as BHA (butylated hydroxyanisole), BHT (butylated hydroxytoluene), TBHQ (tertiary butylhydroquinone)

Guidelines

- Wait two hours after you wake up to eat your breakfast. You can't have anything to eat within two hours of going to sleep.
- You are allowed 1 glass of wine every other day this week. You can substitute a lite beer for the wine, but you can't have both.
- You must drink 1 full cup water before starting to eat each meal.
- Beverages to consume during your feeding window: you can have fresh juice (1 cup per day), 2 cups herbal tea (unsweetened), unlimited plain water (still or fizzy), or water with freshly squeezed citrus like lemon or lime.
- You can have some or all of the following: 1 cup freshly squeezed lemonade per day, 2 cups 1% or 2% milk (soy, low-fat, skim, reduced-fat, coconut), 2 cups coffee per day (each coffee must be 50 calories or less).
- If a sandwich calls for cheese, note that it should be 1 slice of cheese of your choice and the size should be approximately 3½ inches square, which is the typical size of packaged cheese.
- NO white bread (100% whole-grain or 100% whole-wheat bread allowed) or products made with white flour.
- NO soda (regular or diet).
- NO donuts, cake, brownies, pastries, muffins.

- NO creamy salad dressings or sauces.
- NO white potatoes.
- NO frying.

Breakfast Options

- Chia seed pudding with fresh berries and a spoonful of almond butter
- 1½ cups oatmeal with optional 1% or 2% milk, fruit, and 1 teaspoon brown sugar
- 2 pancakes (5 inches in diameter) with 1 slice of bacon and 1 tablespoon 100% maple syrup
- 6-ounce low-fat or fat-free plain Greek yogurt with berries and granola
- 1½ cups cold cereal (7 grams or less sugar per serving) with 1% or 2% milk
- Citrus salad: Slice ½ grapefruit and ½ orange into rounds and arrange on a plate. Scoop 2 tablespoons low-fat or fat-free plain yogurt on top and drizzle with 2 teaspoons organic honey.
- Avocado toast with 100% whole-grain or 100% whole-wheat bread
- 1½ cups Cream of Wheat or farina with optional 1% or 2% milk, fruit, and 1 teaspoon brown sugar
- Veggie hash: Cook 100 grams each of cooked sweet potato, kale, cooked lentils, mushrooms, and bell peppers in a skillet over medium heat for 5 to 10 minutes. Top with chipotle sauce and kelp granules.
- 2 waffles (5 inches in diameter) with 1 slice of bacon and 1 tablespoon 100% maple syrup

- Fruit plate consisting of 4 different fruits
- 12-ounce smoothie
- 12-ounce protein shake
- Avocado and smoked salmon toast (1 toasted slice of 100% whole-grain or 100% whole-wheat bread, ½ small avocado smashed in a bowl with a pinch of cayenne pepper, 2 tablespoons fresh lemon juice, and 2 tablespoons low-fat or fat-free plain yogurt, topped with 3 ounces smoked salmon and cucumber slices, with salt and pepper to taste)
- Egg scramble with 2 eggs and diced veggies and a slice of cheese 3½ inches square
- Breakfast salad: 2 cups mixed greens, ¼ cup blueberries, ¼ cup sliced strawberries, ¼ cup walnuts, and ¼ cup blackberries with 2 tablespoons lemon vinaigrette

Lunch Options

- Quinoa bowl with roasted carrots and sweet potatoes
- Black bean soup with a small green garden salad
- Tomato sandwich with pesto and a drizzle of olive oil and a serving of vegetables
- 5-ounce veggie burger on 100% whole-grain or 100% whole-wheat bread with a small green garden salad
- Tomato basil soup with oyster crackers and a small green garden salad
- Cauliflower rice bowl with black beans, corn, avocado, and salsa
- Easy macro bowl: Use a base of quinoa topped with kale, roasted sweet potato, roasted Brussels sprouts, baked tofu,

kidney beans, tahini, salt, pepper, and lemon juice. Mix and match your choice of grain, legume, and veggies to create your own macro bowl.

- Mediterranean veggie sandwich with a small salad (for the sandwich, use herbed white bean dip or hummus on 100% whole-grain or 100% whole-wheat bread)

- Large green salad (all or any: lettuce, 5 olives, 3 tablespoons shredded cheese, 5 cherry tomatoes, 2 tablespoons nuts, sliced cucumbers) with 2 tablespoons low-fat or fat-free vinaigrette-type dressing and 3 ounces sliced chicken or ½ cup beans if desired; no bacon bits and no croutons

- 1½ cups lentil soup with a small green garden salad

- 2 slices of small cheese pizza (no larger than 4 inches across the crust and 6 inches long) with 1 serving of vegetables

- Tuna avocado salad: Drain 1 can water-packed tuna and combine in a mixing bowl with 2 teaspoons fresh lemon juice, ¼ avocado (mashed), a pinch of salt, and pepper. Scoop the mixture onto a bed of 2 cups leafy greens, cherry tomatoes, ¼ cup red onion slices, and ¼ cup sliced carrots.

- Peanut butter chicken sandwich: Spread 1 tablespoon organic peanut butter on a slice of 100% whole-wheat or 100% whole-grain bread, then top with 4 tablespoons shredded cooked chicken, 1 teaspoon fresh basil, a pinch of salt, and drizzle with extra-virgin olive oil.

Dinner Options

- Veggie stir-fry with tofu
- Cauliflower "steak" with baked sweet potatoes

- Whole-wheat pasta with roasted tomatoes and zucchini or broccoli or both in a marinara or wine sauce
- Vegetarian chili topped with slices of avocado
- Vegetable teriyaki stir-fry
- Black bean tortilla soup with a green garden salad
- 1½ cups soup (no potatoes, no cream). Good choices are chicken noodle, vegetable, lentil, chickpea, split pea, black bean, tomato bisque, etc. Be careful of sodium content. Try for low sodium: 140 mg or less per serving.
- Large green salad (all or any of the following: lettuce, 5 olives, 3 tablespoons shredded cheese, 5 cherry tomatoes, 2 tablespoons nuts, sliced cucumbers) with 2 tablespoons low-fat or fat-free vinaigrette-type dressing and 3 ounces sliced chicken or ½ cup beans if desired; no bacon bits and no croutons
- Green bean and artichoke stir-fry (see recipe, page 271)
- 4 servings of steamed vegetables and 1 cup brown rice
- Chicken burger on a 100% whole-wheat bun with lettuce, tomato, and cheese optional and a small green garden salad
- Spinach turkey salad: In a bowl, mix 3 cups baby spinach, ⅓ cup mushrooms, 1 chopped hard-boiled egg, 2 tablespoons chopped red onion, ¼ cup pecan or walnut halves, 1 small minced clove garlic, and ¼ cup dried cranberries, then top with 4 ounces sliced turkey.
- Broccoli cheddar quesadilla: Place a 10-inch whole-wheat tortilla in a skillet over medium heat, spread cooked broccoli over the tortilla, top with 3 tablespoons shredded cheddar cheese and fold over. Cook on both sides until cheese melts and tortilla is golden brown.

Exercise

Your exercises for each day are listed below. We need to keep ramping up the exercises to keep your body burning fat. I have added some advanced exercises that you can do at home and that don't require any equipment. You can also do them in a gym. All you need is floor space. Please check chapter 13 for instructions on how to do these exercises. You can also find lots of online videos that can show you how to perform the exercises correctly.

DAY 1

30 minutes. Choose a combination of the items below to fulfill your exercise requirement.

Gym Options

- 15 minutes of walking/running on treadmill
- 15 minutes on elliptical machine
- 15 minutes on stationary bicycle
- 15 minutes of swimming laps
- 15 minutes on stair climber
- 15 minutes of spinning
- 15 minutes on rowing machine
- 20 minutes of treadmill intervals

Non-gym Options

- 10 sets of butt kicks (35 seconds of exercise followed by 35 seconds of rest is considered 1 set)
- 10 sets of line hops (35 seconds of exercise followed by 35 seconds of rest is considered 1 set)
- 15 minutes of jogging outside
- 225 jump rope revolutions
- 15 minutes of brisk walking
- 15 minutes of walking up and down a staircase of at least 10 stairs; walking up and down the staircase is considered 1 set (rest between sets as needed)
- 15 minutes of Zumba
- 15 minutes of riding bicycle outside
- 15 minutes of hiking
- 15 minutes of any other high-intensity cardio
- 15 minutes of alternating between running and walking.

Run for 1 minute, then walk for 1 minute, then run again and walk again. Repeat the cycle for 15 minutes.

- 10 sets of jog punches (45 seconds of active exercise followed by 30 seconds of rest is considered 1 set)

Advanced: Note that doing the exercises as described below will fulfill a 15-minute exercise commitment, even if it doesn't take 15 minutes to complete them. In fact, in most cases, you can finish them in half that time depending on your level of conditioning and how aggressive you are.

- 3 sets of squat jumps (10 consecutive jumps per set)
- 5 sets of mountain climbers (30 seconds of continuous exercise followed by 35 seconds of rest is considered 1 set)
- 3 sets of box jumps (10 consecutive jumps per set)
- 3 sets of tuck jumps (10 consecutive jumps per set)
- 5 sets of ice skaters (35 seconds of exercises followed by 35 seconds of rest is considered 1 set)
- 3 sets of jumping lunges (10 consecutive jumps per set)

| | | | | | | | | | | | | | | **DAY 2** | | | | | | | | | | | | | | | |

30 minutes. Choose a combination of the items below to fulfill your exercise requirement.

Gym Options
- 15 minutes of walking/running on treadmill
- 15 minutes on elliptical machine
- 15 minutes on stationary bicycle
- 15 minutes of swimming laps
- 15 minutes on stair climber
- 15 minutes of spinning
- 15 minutes on rowing machine
- 20 minutes treadmill intervals

Non-gym Options
- 10 sets of butt kicks (35 seconds of exercise followed by 35 seconds of rest is considered 1 set)
- 10 sets of line hops (35 seconds of exercise followed by 35 seconds of rest is considered 1 set)
- 15 minutes of jogging outside
- 225 jump rope revolutions
- 15 minutes of brisk walking
- 15 minutes of walking up and down a staircase of at least 10 stairs; walking up and down the staircase is considered 1 set (rest between sets as needed)
- 15 minutes of Zumba
- 15 minutes of riding bicycle outside
- 15 minutes of hiking
- 15 minutes of any other high-intensity cardio
- 15 minutes of alternating between running and walking.

Run for 1 minute, then walk for 1 minute, then run again and walk again. Repeat the cycle for 15 minutes.

- 10 sets of jog punches (45 seconds of active exercise followed by 30 seconds of rest is considered 1 set)

Advanced: Note that doing the exercises as described below will fulfill a 15-minute exercise commitment, even if it doesn't take 15 minutes to complete them. In fact, in most cases, you can finish them in half that time depending on your level of conditioning and how aggressive you are.

- 3 sets of squat jumps (10 consecutive jumps per set)
- 5 sets of mountain climbers (30 seconds of continuous exercise followed by 35 seconds of rest is considered 1 set)
- 3 sets of box jumps (10 consecutive jumps per set)
- 3 sets of tuck jumps (10 consecutive jumps per set)
- 5 sets of ice skaters (35 seconds of exercises followed by 35 seconds of rest is considered 1 set)
- 3 sets of jumping lunges (10 consecutive jumps per set)

DAY 3

- 12,000 steps throughout the day. Use your wearable device or smartphone to keep track.

||||||||||||||||| **DAY 4** |||||||||||||||||||||

30 minutes. Choose a combination of the items below to fulfill your exercise requirement:

Gym Options

- 15 minutes of walking/running on treadmill
- 15 minutes on elliptical machine
- 15 minutes on stationary bicycle
- 15 minutes of swimming laps
- 15 minutes on stair climber
- 15 minutes of spinning
- 15 minutes on rowing machine
- 20 minutes of treadmill intervals

Non-gym Options

- 10 sets of butt kicks (35 seconds of exercise followed by 35 seconds of rest is considered 1 set)
- 10 sets of line hops (35 seconds of exercise followed by 35 seconds of rest is considered 1 set)
- 15 minutes of jogging outside
- 225 jump rope revolutions
- 15 minutes of brisk walking
- 15 minutes of walking up and down a staircase of at least 10 stairs; walking up and down the staircase is considered 1 set (rest between sets as needed)
- 15 minutes of Zumba
- 15 minutes of riding bicycle outside
- 15 minutes of hiking
- 15 minutes of any other high-intensity cardio
- 15 minutes of alternating between running and walking.

Run for 1 minute, then walk for 1 minute, then run again and walk again. Repeat the cycle for 15 minutes.

- 10 sets of jog punches (45 seconds of active exercise followed by 30 seconds of rest is considered 1 set)

Advanced: Note that doing the exercises as described below will fulfill a 15-minute exercise commitment, even if it doesn't take 15 minutes to complete them. In fact, in most cases, you can finish them in half that time depending on your level of conditioning and how aggressive you are.

- 3 sets of squat jumps (10 consecutive jumps per set)
- 5 sets of mountain climbers (30 seconds of continuous exercise followed by 35 seconds of rest is considered 1 set)
- 3 sets of box jumps (10 consecutive jumps per set)
- 3 sets of tuck jumps (10 consecutive jumps per set)
- 5 sets of ice skaters (35 seconds of exercises followed by 35 seconds of rest is considered 1 set)
- 3 sets of jumping lunges (10 consecutive jumps per set)

DAY 5

30 minutes. Choose a combination of the items below to fulfill your exercise requirement:

Gym Options

- 15 minutes of walking/running on treadmill
- 15 minutes on elliptical machine
- 15 minutes on stationary bicycle
- 15 minutes of swimming laps
- 15 minutes on stair climber
- 15 minutes of spinning
- 15 minutes on rowing machine
- 20 minutes of treadmill intervals

Non-gym Options

- 10 sets of butt kicks (35 seconds of exercise followed by 35 seconds of rest is considered 1 set)
- 10 sets of line hops (35 seconds of exercise followed by 35 seconds of rest is considered 1 set)
- 15 minutes of jogging outside
- 225 jump rope revolutions
- 15 minutes of brisk walking
- 15 minutes of walking up and down a staircase of at least 10 stairs; walking up and down the staircase is considered 1 set (rest between sets as needed)
- 15 minutes of Zumba
- 15 minutes of riding bicycle outside
- 15 minutes of hiking
- 15 minutes of any other high-intensity cardio
- 15 minutes of alternating between running and walking.

Run for 1 minute, then walk for 1 minute, then run again and walk again. Repeat the cycle for 15 minutes.

- 10 sets of jog punches (45 seconds of active exercise followed by 30 seconds of rest is considered 1 set)

Advanced: Note that doing the exercises as described below will fulfill a 15-minute exercise commitment, even if it doesn't take 15 minutes to complete them. In fact, in most cases, you can finish them in half that time depending on your level of conditioning and how aggressive you are.

- 3 sets of squat jumps (10 consecutive jumps per set)
- 5 sets of mountain climbers (30 seconds of continuous exercise followed by 35 seconds of rest is considered 1 set)
- 3 sets of box jumps (10 consecutive jumps per set)
- 3 sets of tuck jumps (10 consecutive jumps per set)
- 5 sets of ice skaters (35 seconds of exercises followed by 35 seconds of rest is considered 1 set)
- 3 sets of jumping lunges (10 consecutive jumps per set)

DAY 6

Rest day

| | | | | | | | | | | | | | | | | **DAY 7** | | | | | | | | | | | | | | | |

- 14,000 steps throughout the day. Use your wearable device or smartphone to keep track.
- 15 sets of stairs (up and down at least 10 steps is considered 1 set).

10

Week 8:

Stretch

YOU'RE ENTERING THE SECOND-TO-LAST WEEK OF THIS awesome journey. I know it hasn't been the easiest thing you've ever done, but the fact that you are here means that in many ways you've already been successful. Now is the time for you to prepare to go all out. Think about the great marathoners at the end of a long race. Somehow, despite having run over twenty miles, they're able to summon enough energy to stretch their legs and increase their stride as they race toward the finish line. They pick up the pace before they can actually see the finishing tape. Next week you will be able to see the tape, but this week, you have to trust that the end is near. Now is the time you must summon the strength to go faster, despite all the fatigue, aches in your muscles, and burn in your lungs.

There's no holding back when you're close to finishing. The next two weeks will ask you to put it all on the table. You've gotten through seven weeks, surely you can get through the next two. This week is particularly different, so make sure you pay attention to all of the guidelines and the specific instructions in the daily meal plans. You will be eating only two meals each day with four snacks. Three of these snacks must come between the meals and the last snack must come after dinner. It's important that you follow the schedule as written to maximize the success of the week.

For this week and the last, we are going to do something very different with the IF schedule. For those who want to be the most aggressive, you will move to 16:8 fasting/feeding windows. For example, you might decide to start your fasting window at 8 P.M. and run it all the way to 12 P.M. the next day. Your feeding window would run from 12 P.M. to 8 P.M. For those who don't want to be as aggressive, you should follow the 14:10 schedule. For example, you might start your fasting window at 8 P.M. and end it at 10 A.M. You would then eat your meals and snacks between 10 A.M. and 8 P.M.

We are going to do something else a little different these last two weeks. You will also be following a 5:2 IF schedule, which means that five of the days you will be eating almost double the calories you'll be eating on two low-calorie days. I'm calling this a **Daily Double**. This will be a bit of a challenge for some, as it's very different from what you've been doing, but trust that you will not just get through it, but you will thrive and achieve strong results. If you simply don't have the appetite to increase your calories by the amount allowed in the meal plan, don't worry about it. Simply eat what satisfies you. Never eat when you're not hungry just because the plan calls for a meal or snack or a certain volume of food. I tried this combined IF strategy with thousands of my followers on social media, and there was a noticeable spike in their results. Many lost a significant amount of weight, while others who had plateaued finally started to see the scale move again. Look at the entire week's meal plan in advance. Make sure you map out the foods you will need, as well as when and where you will be able to eat them. Preparation for these last two weeks is critical to helping you conquer them with greater ease and confidence.

You're also going to have a bonus snack in the event that you really need it. This is called a **Floating Bonus Snack**. It should not exceed 100 calories. The purpose of this snack is like an emergency life-line. When you feel like you really need some energy and nutrients, something to get you through when your stomach is growling and you just need that little infusion to make it. If you don't need or want it, simply don't eat it. Don't force yourself to eat it just because it's available.

Guidelines

- Set your fasting/feeding windows and stick to them for the entire week.
- Your low-calorie days have reduced exercise, so be mindful of that.
- Try to make sure you space your snacks at least an hour apart, and the last one should be at least an hour after you finish dinner.
- 1 glass of wine or 1 lite beer is allowed every other day, except for the low-calorie days.
- If a sandwich calls for cheese, note that it should be 1 slice of cheese of your choice and the size should be approximately 3½ inches square, which is the typical size of packaged cheese.
- No soda.
- No frying.
- Each day you're allowed an extra snack of 100 calories or less if you really need it. This is called your **Floating Bonus Snack!**
- Try one of the new exercises added to the exercise options.

| | | | | | | | | | | | | | **DAY 1** | | | | | | | | | | | | | | |

Meal 1

- 1 piece of fruit. Choose from the following, though you can choose others: pear, apple, ½ cup raspberries or strawberries or blueberries or blackberries, ½ grapefruit, ½ cup cherries.

Choose one of the following:

- 2 pancakes (5 inches in diameter) with 1 slice of bacon and 1 tablespoon 100% maple syrup
- 2 scrambled eggs (diced veggies and 3 tablespoons shredded cheese or 1 slice of cheese 3½ inches square optional; a little butter or cooking spray allowed)
- 1 egg white omelet (2 egg whites or ½ cup Egg Beaters; diced veggies optional)
- 1 cup oatmeal
- 1 cup cold cereal (7 g or less sugar) with 1% or 2% milk

Beverages

- You can have 1 cup fresh juice (not from concentrate) *or* 1 cup 1% or 2% milk, or unsweetened soy or almond milk.
- You can have 1 cup coffee (50 calories or less) or 1 cup herbal tea along with the juice or milk.
- **Optional**: unlimited plain water or water with freshly squeezed citrus like lemon or lime.

Eat your snacks 90 to 100 minutes after your meal!

Snack 1

- ½ cup roasted pumpkin seeds *or* 10 baked whole-wheat pita chips *or* any other item 150 calories or less

Snack 2

- 1½ cups puffed rice *or* 1 cup broccoli florets with 2 tablespoons dip *or* any other item 100 calories or less

Snack 3

- Any item 150 calories or less

Meal 2

- Choose one of the following:
- 6-ounce piece of chicken (baked or grilled, no skin) with 2 servings of vegetables
- Grilled chicken salad (lettuce, cucumbers, cherry tomatoes, ½ sliced avocado, 2 tablespoons feta cheese, 5 ounces sliced grilled chicken)
- 6-ounce piece of turkey (baked or grilled, no skin) with 2 servings of vegetables
- 6-ounce piece of fish (baked or grilled) with 2 servings of vegetables

Beverages

Choose one of the following. In addition to your choice you can have unlimited plain flat or fizzy water.

- 1 cup flavored water
- 1 cup freshly squeezed lemonade
- 1 cup unsweetened iced tea
- 1 cup juice (not from concentrate)
- 1 cup 1% or 2% milk or unsweetened soy or almond milk

Snack 4

- Any item 100 calories or less

Exercise

40 minutes. Choose a combination of the items below to fulfill your exercise requirement:

Gym Options

- 15 minutes of walking/running on treadmill
- 15 minutes on elliptical machine
- 15 minutes on stationary bicycle
- 15 minutes of swimming laps
- 15 minutes on stair climber
- 15 minutes of spinning
- 15 minutes on rowing machine
- 20 minutes of treadmill intervals

Non-gym Options

- 5 sets of running high knees (35 seconds of running followed by 35 seconds of rest is considered 1 set)
- 4 sets of stationary squats (15 squats per set)
- 10 sets of butt kicks (35 seconds of exercise followed by 35 seconds of rest is considered 1 set)
- 10 sets of line hops (35 seconds of exercise followed by 35 seconds of rest is considered 1 set)
- 15 minutes of jogging outside
- 225 jump rope revolutions
- 15 minutes of brisk walking
- 15 minutes of walking up and down a staircase of at least 10 stairs; walking up and down the staircase is considered 1 set (rest between sets as needed)
- 15 minutes of Zumba
- 15 minutes of riding bicycle outside
- 15 minutes of hiking
- 15 minutes of any other high-intensity cardio
- 15 minutes of alternating between running and walking. Run for 1 minute, then walk for 1 minute, then run again and walk again. Repeat the cycle for 15 minutes.

- 10 sets of jog punches (45 seconds of active exercise followed by 30 seconds of rest is considered 1 set)

Advanced: Note that doing the exercises as described below will fulfill a 15-minute exercise commitment, even if it doesn't take 15 minutes to complete them. In fact, in most cases, you can finish them in half that time depending on your level of conditioning and how aggressive you are.

- 3 sets of squat jumps (10 consecutive jumps per set)
- 5 sets of mountain climbers (30 seconds of continuous exercise followed by 35 seconds of rest is considered 1 set)
- 3 sets of box jumps (10 consecutive jumps per set)
- 3 sets of tuck jumps (10 consecutive jumps per set)
- 5 sets of ice skaters (35 seconds of exercises followed by 35 seconds of rest is considered 1 set)
- 3 sets of jumping lunges (10 consecutive jumps per set)

DAY 2

Meal 1

Choose one of the following:

- 1 cup cooked oatmeal with optional 1% or 2% milk, fruit, and ½ teaspoon brown sugar
- 1 cup Cream of Wheat or farina with optional 1% or 2% milk, fruit, and ½ teaspoon brown sugar
- 1 cup cold cereal (7 g or less sugar) with 1% or 2% milk
- 6-ounce low-fat or fat-free plain Greek yogurt with fresh fruit
- Baked Apple Heaven (see recipe, page 255)

Beverages

- You can have 1 cup fresh juice (not from concentrate) *or* 1 cup 1% or 2% milk, or unsweetened soy or almond milk.
- You can have 1 cup coffee (50 calories or less) or 1 cup herbal tea along with the juice or milk.
- **Optional**: unlimited plain water or water with freshly squeezed citrus like lemon or lime

Snack 1

- 5 crackers *or* ½ blueberry muffin *or* any snack item 150 calories or less

Snack 2

- 10 baby carrots with 2 tablespoons low-fat hummus *or* ½ frozen banana dipped in chocolate *or* any snack item 100 calories or less

Snack 3

- Any item 150 calories or less

Meal 2

Choose one of the following:

- 2 slices of small cheese pizza (no larger than 4 inches across the crust and 6 inches long) with 2 servings of vegetables
- 1 serving of lasagna (with or without meat), 4 by 3 by 1 inch.
- Steak salad (6 ounces thinly sliced steak over a bed of 2 cups
- arugula, plum tomato cut into wedges, 1 sliced scallion, ⅓ cup sliced pineapple, and 1 tablespoon fresh lime juice)
- 6-ounce veggie burger with 2 servings of vegetables
- 6 ounces turkey or chicken (grilled or baked, no skin, not fried) with 2 servings of vegetables

Beverages

Choose one of the following. Regardless of your choice, you can have unlimited plain flat or fizzy water.

- 1 cup flavored water
- 1 cup freshly squeezed lemonade
- 1 cup unsweetened iced tea
- 1 cup juice (not from concentrate)
- 1 cup 1% or 2% milk or unsweetened soy or almond milk

Snack 4

- 2 ounces smoked salmon *or* 6 oysters *or* any snack item 100 calories or less

Exercise

30 minutes. Choose 2 of the following exercises for a total of 30 minutes:

Gym Options

- 15 minutes of walking/running on treadmill

- 15 minutes on elliptical machine
- 15 minutes on stationary bicycle
- 15 minutes of swimming laps
- 15 minutes on stair climber
- 15 minutes of spinning
- 15 minutes on rowing machine
- 20 minutes of treadmill intervals

Non-gym Options

- 5 sets of running high knees (35 seconds of running followed by 35 seconds of rest is considered 1 set)
- 4 sets of stationary squats (15 squats per set)
- 10 sets of butt kicks (35 seconds of exercise followed by 35 seconds of rest is considered 1 set)
- 10 sets of line hops (35 seconds of exercise followed by 35 seconds of rest is considered 1 set)
- 15 minutes of jogging outside
- 225 jump rope revolutions
- 15 minutes of brisk walking
- 15 minutes of walking up and down a staircase of at least 10 stairs; walking up and down the staircase is considered 1 set (rest between sets as needed)
- 15 minutes of Zumba
- 15 minutes of riding bicycle outside
- 15 minutes of hiking
- 15 minutes of any other high-intensity cardio
- 15 minutes of alternating between running and walking. Run for 1 minute, then walk for 1 minute, then run again and walk again. Repeat the cycle for 15 minutes.

- 10 sets of jog punches (45 seconds of active exercise followed by 30 seconds of rest is considered 1 set)

Advanced: Note that doing the exercises as described below will fulfill a 15-minute exercise commitment, even if it doesn't take 15 minutes to complete them. In fact, in most cases, you can finish them in half that time depending on your level of conditioning and how aggressive you are.

- 3 sets of squat jumps (10 consecutive jumps per set)
- 5 sets of mountain climbers (30 seconds of continuous exercise followed by 35 seconds of rest is considered 1 set)
- 3 sets of box jumps (10 consecutive jumps per set)
- 3 sets of tuck jumps (10 consecutive jumps per set)
- 5 sets of ice skaters (35 seconds of exercises followed by 35 seconds of rest is considered 1 set)
- 3 sets of jumping lunges (10 consecutive jumps per set)

| | | | | | | DAY 3 (Low-Calorie Day) | | | | | | |

NOTE: Don't forget that you're allowed a **Floating Bonus Snack** today!

Meal 1

Choose one of the following. Make sure it's 200 calories or less; no sugar added.

- 12-ounce fruit smoothie (250 calories or less; no sugar added)
- 12-ounce protein shake (250 calories or less; no sugar added)
- 8-ounce yogurt parfait

Beverages

- You can have 1 cup fresh juice (not from concentrate) *or* 1 cup coffee that's 50 calories or less.
- You can have unlimited plain water, flat or fizzy, or water with freshly squeezed citrus like lemon or lime

Snack 1

- 1 cup grape tomatoes *or* ½ cup roasted chickpeas *or* any other item 100 calories or less

Snack 2

- Hard-boiled egg with ½ cup sugar snap peas *or* ½ cup fat-free yogurt and ½ cup blueberries *or* any other item 100 calories or less

Snack 3

- 1 medium cucumber sprinkled with balsamic vinaigrette *or* 9 or 10 black olives *or* any other item 100 calories or less

Meal 2

- 1 cup soup (no potatoes, no cream). Good choices are chicken noodle, vegetable, lentil, chickpea, split pea, black bean, tomato basil, minestrone. Always be careful of sodium content! Try for low sodium: 140 mg or less per serving.
- ½ cup brown rice
- 1 serving of vegetables
- Cheesy whole-wheat pasta (1 cup cooked whole-wheat fusilli pasta topped with 1 cup chopped broccoli florets and 3 tablespoons shredded organic Parmesan, with salt and pepper to taste)

Beverages

Choose one of the following:

- Unlimited plain water (flat or fizzy) or water with freshly squeezed citrus like lemon or lime
- 1 cup flavored water
- 1 cup freshly squeezed lemonade
- 1 cup unsweetened iced tea

Exercise

Rest day

| | | | | | | | | | | | | | | **DAY 4** | | | | | | | | | | | | | | | |

Meal 1

- 12-ounce fruit smoothie (300 calories or less; no added sugar)
- 12-ounce protein shake (300 calories or less; no added sugar)

Snack 1

- 2 stalks celery and 2 ounces hummus *or* 8 baby carrot sticks (or 20 cucumber slices) and 2 ounces of hummus *or* 1 small baked sweet potato with 2 tablespoons fat-free sour cream or ½ teaspoon butter *or* any item 150 calories or less

Snack 2

- 2 cups air-popped popcorn with small amount of salt *or* 1 fat-free chocolate or vanilla pudding *or* 1½ cups sugar snap peas *or* any item 150 calories or less

Snack 3

- 1 hard-boiled egg (lightly salt and pepper to taste) *or* 15 olives *or* 1 cup mixed raw vegetables with 1 tablespoon balsamic vinaigrette

Meal 2

- 1½ cups soup (no potatoes, no cream) with a small salad. Good choices are vegetable, lentil, chickpea, split pea, black bean, tomato bisque, etc. Be careful of sodium content. Try for low sodium: 140 mg or less per serving. Try the Luscious Pea Soup (see recipe, page 263).
- Large green salad (all or any of the following: lettuce, 5 olives, 3 tablespoons shredded cheese, 5 cherry tomatoes, 2 tablespoons nuts, sliced cucumbers) with

2 tablespoons low-fat or fat-free vinaigrette-type dressing and 3 ounces sliced chicken or ½ cup beans if desired; no bacon bits and no croutons

- Tuna avocado salad: Drain 1 can water-packed tuna and combine in a mixing bowl with 2 teaspoons fresh lemon juice, ¼ avocado (mashed), a pinch of salt, and pepper. Scoop the mixture onto a bed of 2 cups leafy greens, cherry tomatoes, ¼ cup red onion slices, and ¼ cup sliced carrots.

Snack 4

- 20 raw almonds or 15 cashews *or* 1 medium banana and 1 tablespoon cottage cheese *or* any item 100 calories or less

Exercise

Rest day. However, if you want to push yourself, 10,000 steps.

DAY 5

Meal 1

Choose one of the following:

- 1 cup oatmeal with optional 1% or 2% milk, fruit, and 1 teaspoon brown sugar
- 1 cup Cream of Wheat or farina with optional 1% or 2% milk, fruit, and 1 teaspoon brown sugar
- 1 cup cold cereal (7 g or less sugar) with 1% or 2% milk and 1 serving of fruit

Beverages

- You can have 1 cup fresh juice (not from concentrate) *or* 1 cup 1% or 2% milk, or unsweetened soy or almond milk.
- You can have 1 cup coffee (50 calories or less) or 1 cup herbal tea along with the juice or milk.
- **Optional**: unlimited plain water or water with freshly squeezed citrus like lemon or lime

Snack 1

- Any item 150 calories or less.

Snack 2

- Any item 150 calories or less

Snack 3

- Any item 150 calories or less

Meal 2

Choose one of the following:

- 1 cup soup (no potatoes, no cream). Good choices are chicken noodle, vegetable, lentil, chickpea, split pea, black bean, tomato basil, minestrone. Always be careful of sodium content! Try for low sodium: 140 mg or less per serving.

- Tomato pesto pasta (1 cup cooked whole-wheat penne pasta with 5 halved cherry tomatoes cooked in a skillet in olive oil until soft and 2 tablespoons pesto)
- Large green salad (all or any: lettuce, 5 olives, 3 tablespoons shredded cheese, 5 cherry tomatoes, 2 tablespoons nuts, sliced cucumbers) with 2 tablespoons low-fat or fat-free vinaigrette-type dressing and 3 ounces sliced chicken or ½ cup beans if desired; no bacon bits and no croutons
- 6 ounces of baked or grilled chicken or fish with 2 servings of vegetables

Beverages

Choose one of the following. Regardless of your choice, you can have unlimited plain flat or fizzy water.

- 1 cup flavored water
- 1 cup freshly squeezed lemonade
- 1 cup unsweetened iced tea
- 1 cup juice (not from concentrate)
- 1 cup 1% or 2% milk or unsweetened soy or almond milk

Snack 4

- Any item 100 calories or less

Exercise

30 minutes of cardio. Choose a combination of the items below to fulfill your exercise requirement.

Gym Options

- 15 minutes of walking/running on treadmill
- 15 minutes on elliptical machine
- 15 minutes on stationary bicycle

- 15 minutes of swimming laps
- 15 minutes on stair climber
- 15 minutes of spinning
- 15 minutes on rowing machine
- 20 minutes of treadmill intervals

Non-gym Options

- 5 sets of running high knees (35 seconds of running followed by 35 seconds of rest is considered 1 set)
- 4 sets of stationary squats (15 squats per set)
- 10 sets of butt kicks (35 seconds of exercise followed by 35 seconds of rest is considered 1 set)
- 10 sets of line hops (35 seconds of exercise followed by 35 seconds of rest is considered 1 set)
- 15 minutes of jogging outside
- 225 jump rope revolutions
- 15 minutes of brisk walking
- 15 minutes of walking up and down a staircase of at least 10 stairs; walking up and down the staircase is considered 1 set (rest between sets as needed)
- 15 minutes of Zumba
- 15 minutes of riding bicycle outside
- 15 minutes of hiking
- 15 minutes of any other high-intensity cardio
- 15 minutes of alternating between running and walking. Run for 1 minute, then walk for 1 minute, then run again and walk again. Repeat the cycle for 15 minutes.
- 10 sets of jog punches (45 seconds of active exercise followed by 30 seconds of rest is considered 1 set)

Advanced

Doing the exercises as described below will fulfill a 15-minute exercise commitment, even if it doesn't take 15 minutes to complete them. In fact, in most cases, you can finish them in half that time depending on your level of conditioning and how aggressive you are.

- 3 sets of squat jumps (10 consecutive jumps per set)
- 5 sets of mountain climbers (30 seconds of continuous exercise followed by 35 seconds of rest is considered 1 set)
- 3 sets of box jumps (10 consecutive jumps per set)
- 3 sets of tuck jumps (10 consecutive jumps per set)
- 5 sets of ice skaters (35 seconds of exercises followed by 35 seconds of rest is considered 1 set)
- 3 sets of jumping lunges (10 consecutive jumps per set)

DAY 6 (Low-Calorie Day)

NOTE: Don't forget that you're allowed a **Floating Bonus Snack** today!

Meal 1
Choose one of the following:
- 12-ounce fruit smoothie (250 calories or less, no added sugar)
- 12-ounce protein shake (250 calories or less, no added sugar)
- 8-ounce yogurt parfait

Beverages
Optional: unlimited plain water or water with freshly squeezed citrus like lemon or lime
Optional: 1 cup coffee (no more than 1 packet sugar and 1 tablespoon milk or half-and-half) or 1 cup herbal tea

Snack 1
- 1 cup grape tomatoes *or* 1½ cups fruit salad *or* any snack item 100 calories or less

Snack 2
- 8 small shrimp with 3 tablespoons cocktail sauce *or* ½ cup low-fat salsa with 10 tortilla chips *or* any snack item 100 calories or less

Snack 3
- 4 chocolate chip cookies the size of a poker chip *or* ½ cup roasted chickpeas *or* any snack item 100 calories or less

Meal 2
Choose one of the following. Make sure it is different from yesterday's second meal.

- 6-ounce piece of chicken (baked or grilled, no skin) with 2 servings of vegetables
- Shrimp salad: Cook 4 shrimp in a skillet over medium heat, then add ½ cup corn and ½ cup black beans, salt, and pepper. Cook for 3 to 5 minutes, then serve.
- 6-ounce piece of turkey (baked or grilled, no skin) with 2 servings of vegetables
- 6-ounce piece of fish (baked or grilled) with 2 servings of vegetables
- Large green garden salad (3 cups greens) with 3 ounces sliced chicken. You may include a few olives, shredded carrots, ½ sliced tomato or 5 grape tomatoes, and sliced cucumbers. Only 2 tablespoons fat-free or low-fat vinaigrette-style dressing. No bacon bits, no croutons.
- 1 cup whole-grain pasta with marinara sauce (ground meat optional)

Beverages

Choose one of the following:

- Unlimited plain water (flat or fizzy) or water with freshly squeezed citrus like lemon or lime
- 1 cup flavored water
- 1 cup freshly squeezed lemonade
- 1 cup unsweetened iced tea
- 1 cup juice (not from concentrate)
- 1 cup 1% or 2% milk or unsweetened soy or almond milk

Snack 4

- Any item 100 calories or less

Exercise

Rest day

DAY 7

Meal 1

Choose one of the following:

- 8-ounce yogurt parfait
- 1 egg-white omelet (made with 2 egg whites or ½ cup Egg Beaters; a little butter or cooking spray is allowed)
- 1 cup cold cereal (7 g or less sugar) with 1% or 2% milk and one serving of fruit

Optional: 1 piece of 100% whole-grain or 100% whole-wheat toast

Beverages

- You can have 1 cup fresh juice (not from concentrate) *or* 1 cup 1% or 2% milk or unsweetened soy or almond milk.
- You can have 1 cup coffee (50 calories or less) along with the juice or milk or 1 cup herbal tea.
- **Optional**: unlimited plain water or water with freshly squeezed citrus like lemon or lime

Snack 1

- Any item 150 calories or less

Snack 2

- 1 medium cucumber sprinkled with balsamic vinaigrette *or* 9 or 10 black olives *or* any other item 100 calories or less

Snack 3

- Any item 150 calories or less

Meal 2

- 1 cup brown rice
- 1 cup cooked beans, chickpeas, or lentils (no baked beans)

- 1 serving of vegetables
- Tomato and peach salad: In a bowl, combine ½ small thinly sliced red onion, 1 teaspoon red wine vinegar, and a pinch of salt. Slice 1 tomato and 1 peach and arrange on a plate. Drizzle the onion mixture over the tomato and peach slices. Add ¼ cup crumbled feta if desired.

Beverages

Choose one of the following. Regardless of your choice, you can have unlimited plain flat or fizzy water.

- 1 cup flavored water
- 1 cup freshly squeezed lemonade
- 1 cup unsweetened iced tea
- 1 cup juice (not from concentrate)
- 1 cup 1% or 2% milk or unsweetened soy or almond milk

Snack 4

- Any item 150 calories or less

Exercise

30 minutes. Choose 2 of the following exercises for a total of 30 minutes:

Gym Options

- 15 minutes of walking/running on treadmill
- 15 minutes on elliptical machine
- 15 minutes on stationary bicycle
- 15 minutes of swimming laps
- 15 minutes on stair climber
- 15 minutes of spinning
- 15 minutes on rowing machine
- 20 minutes of treadmill intervals

Non-gym Options

- 5 sets of running high knees (35 seconds of running followed by 35 seconds of rest is considered 1 set)
- 4 sets of stationary squats (15 squats per set)
- 10 sets of butt kicks (35 seconds of exercise followed by 35 seconds of rest is considered 1 set)
- 10 sets of line hops (35 seconds of exercise followed by 35 seconds of rest is considered 1 set)
- 15 minutes of jogging outside
- 225 jump rope revolutions
- 15 minutes of brisk walking
- 15 minutes of walking up and down a staircase of at least 10 stairs; walking up and down the staircase is considered 1 set (rest between sets as needed)
- 15 minutes of Zumba
- 15 minutes of riding bicycle outside
- 15 minutes of hiking
- 15 minutes of any other high-intensity cardio
- 15 minutes of alternating between running and walking. Run for 1 minute, then walk for 1 minute, then run again and walk again. Repeat the cycle for 15 minutes.
- 10 sets of jog punches (45 seconds of active exercise followed by 30 seconds of rest is considered 1 set)

Advanced

Doing the exercises as described below will fulfill a 15-minute exercise commitment, even if it doesn't take 15 minutes to complete them. In fact, in most cases, you can finish them in half that time depending on your level of conditioning and how aggressive you are.

- 3 sets of squat jumps (10 consecutive jumps per set)
- 5 sets of mountain climbers (30 seconds of continuous exercise followed by 35 seconds of rest is considered 1 set)
- 3 sets of box jumps (10 consecutive jumps per set)
- 3 sets of tuck jumps (10 consecutive jumps per set)
- 5 sets of ice skaters (35 seconds of exercises followed by 35 seconds of rest is considered 1 set)
- 3 sets of jumping lunges (10 consecutive jumps per set)

11

Week 9:

Kick

CONGRATULATIONS ON MAKING IT TO YOUR LAST WEEK! Take a moment to reflect on how far you've come on this journey. While we often direct most of our attention to the scale, it's also important that we give ourselves credit for the non-scale victories (NSV) we've been able to accomplish. This is your week to really go hard and cross the finish line. Now you can finally see the tape at the end of this marathon and it's time to run through it with all that you have. Let these three words be your guide: GET IT DONE!!!

Your IF schedule will be 16:8. For those who are truly ambitious, you can try 18:6. Whichever you choose, it's important that you stick to it for the entire week. At this point you should know what you're cable of and how hard you can push yourself.

Please pay close attention to the details of the meal plan this week and follow it as closely as possible. This is designed to be a very simple and clean week. You must really kick hard this week. Be extra vigilant about choices and portions. Block out all the background noise and distractions and give it absolutely everything you've got. Be proud of yourself regardless of what the scale shows at the end of this week. You may not have been perfect on this journey, but you hung in there and kept getting back up when you fell. For that reason alone, you are a WINNER!

Guidelines

- You choose what you want to do for exercise, as long as you meet the time requirement.

- Drink 1 cup water before every meal! Do not take your first bite until you have finished the entire cup.

- Don't eat your first meal or any solid food until two hours after getting up. Your last solid food must be BEFORE two hours of going to sleep—in other words, nothing to eat within two hours of going to bed.

- Drink 1 cup lemon water—hot or cold—each day. You choose the time.

- No alcohol.

- Organic honey is allowed.

- Organic 100% stevia is allowed.

- Burritos can be homemade or frozen. If you opt for a frozen burrito, make sure it's low in sodium (300 mg or less per serving).

- If a sandwich calls for cheese, note that it should be 1 slice of cheese of your choice and the size should be approximately 3½ inches square, which is the typical size of packaged cheese.

- NO artificial sweeteners.

- NO frying—except to stir-fry veggies in olive oil.

- NO white bread (100% whole-grain or 100% whole-wheat bread allowed).

- NO soda.

- NO white pasta.

| | | | | | | | | | | | | | | **DAY 1** | | | | | | | | | | | | | | | | |

Meal 1

Choose one of the following:

- 2 scrambled eggs with diced veggies and 3 tablespoons shredded cheese or 1 slice of cheese 3½ inches square and 1 serving of fruit

- 1 cup steel-cut oats with optional 1% or 2% milk, fruit, and ½ teaspoon brown sugar

- 1 cup grits with optional 1% or 2% milk, fruit, and ½ teaspoon brown sugar

- 1 cup Cream of Wheat or farina with optional 1% or 2% milk, fruit, and ½ teaspoon brown sugar

- Herbed Egg-White Wraps (see recipe, page 257)

Snack

- Any item 150 calories or less

Meal 2

Choose one of the following:

- Large green garden salad (all or any of the following: lettuce, tomatoes, peppers, 1 hard-boiled egg, ¼ cup chunked avocado, sliced cucumbers) with 2 tablespoons fat-free or low-fat vinaigrette-style dressing

- 1½ cups soup (butternut squash, lentil, black bean, white bean, tomato, or cucumber). Try the Silky Butternut Squash and Apple Soup (see recipe, page 265).

- Peanut butter chicken sandwich: Spread 1 tablespoon organic peanut butter on a slice of 100% whole-wheat or 100% whole-grain bread, then top with 4 tablespoons shredded cooked chicken, 1 teaspoon fresh basil, and a pinch of salt and drizzle with extra-virgin olive oil.

Snack

- Any item 100 calories or less

Meal 3

Choose one of the following:

- 1½ cups whole-grain spaghetti with optional diced zucchini, squash, peppers, tomatoes, and/or broccoli in a marinara or lemon-wine sauce
- 4 servings of vegetables with ½ cup brown rice
- Cheesy Chicken Quesadilla (see page 277)

Snack

- Any item 100 calories or less

Exercise

30 minutes. Choose 2 of the following exercises for a total of 30 minutes:

Gym Options

- 15 minutes of walking/running on treadmill
- 15 minutes on elliptical machine
- 15 minutes on stationary bicycle
- 15 minutes of swimming laps
- 15 minutes on stair climber
- 15 minutes of spinning
- 15 minutes on rowing machine
- 20 minutes of treadmill intervals

Non-gym Options

- 8 sets of frog jumps (10 jumps per set)
- 5 sets of running high knees (35 seconds of running followed by 35 seconds of rest is considered 1 set)
- 4 sets of stationary squats (15 squats per set)

- 10 sets of butt kicks (35 seconds of exercise followed by 35 seconds of rest is considered 1 set)
- 10 sets of line hops (35 seconds of exercise followed by 35 seconds of rest is considered 1 set)
- 15 minutes of jogging outside
- 225 jump rope revolutions
- 15 minutes of brisk walking
- 15 minutes of walking up and down a staircase of at least 10 stairs; walking up and down the staircase is considered 1 set (rest between sets as needed)
- 15 minutes of Zumba
- 15 minutes of riding bicycle outside
- 15 minutes of hiking
- 15 minutes of any other high-intensity cardio
- 15 minutes of alternating between running and walking. Run for 1 minute, then walk for 1 minute, then run again and walk again. Repeat the cycle for 15 minutes.
- 10 sets of jog punches (45 seconds of active exercise followed by 30 seconds of rest is considered 1 set)

Advanced: Note that doing the exercises as described below will fulfill a 15-minute exercise commitment, even if it doesn't take 15 minutes to complete them. In fact, in most cases, you can finish them in half that time depending on your level of conditioning and how aggressive you are.

- 8 sets of plank jacks (10 jacks per set)
- 3 sets of squat jumps (10 consecutive jumps per set)
- 5 sets of mountain climbers (30 seconds of continuous exercise followed by 35 seconds of rest is considered 1 set)
- 3 sets of box jumps (10 consecutive jumps per set)

- 3 sets of tuck jumps (10 consecutive jumps per set)
- 5 sets of ice skaters (35 seconds of exercises followed by 35 seconds of rest is considered 1 set)
- 3 sets of jumping lunges (10 consecutive jumps per set)

| | | | | | | | | | | | | | | | **DAY 2** | | | | | | | | | | | | | | | |

Meal 1

Choose one of the following:

- 8-ounce plain low-fat Greek yogurt with fresh fruit
- 12-ounce fresh fruit smoothie (300 calories or less; no added sugar). Try the Tropical Dash Smoothie (see recipe, page 285).

Snack

- Any item 100 calories or less

Meal 2

Choose one of the following:

- Beef Burrito Bowl (see recipe, page 268)
- Egg salad spread over 1 slice of toasted or untoasted 100% whole-grain or 100% whole-wheat bread (for the egg salad, use 2 whole eggs, low-fat mayo, dill, mustard, chives, salt and pepper)

Snack

- Any item 100 calories or less

Meal 3

Choose one of the following:

- 1½ cups soup (lentil, black bean, white bean, tomato, squash, vegetable, or cucumber)
- 2 small roasted vegetable and black bean tacos (5-inch diameter)
- Cheesy whole-wheat pasta (1 cup cooked whole-wheat fusilli pasta topped with 1 cup chopped broccoli florets and 3 tablespoons shredded organic Parmesan, with salt and pepper to taste)

Snack

- Any item 100 calories or less

Exercise

- 30 minutes. Break up into a morning and afternoon/evening session. Choose 2 of the following exercises for a total of 30 minutes:

Gym Options

- 15 minutes of walking/running on treadmill
- 15 minutes on elliptical machine
- 15 minutes on stationary bicycle
- 15 minutes of swimming laps
- 15 minutes on stair climber
- 15 minutes of spinning
- 15 minutes on rowing machine
- 20 minutes of treadmill intervals

Non-gym Options

- 8 sets of frog jumps (10 jumps per set)
- 5 sets of running high knees (35 seconds of running followed by 35 seconds of rest is considered 1 set)
- 4 sets of stationary squats (15 squats per set)
- 10 sets of butt kicks (35 seconds of exercise followed by 35 seconds of rest is considered 1 set)
- 10 sets of line hops (35 seconds of exercise followed by 35 seconds of rest is considered 1 set)
- 15 minutes of jogging outside
- 225 jump rope revolutions
- 15 minutes of brisk walking
- 15 minutes of walking up and down a staircase of at least

10 stairs; walking up and down the staircase is considered
1 set (rest between sets as needed)

- 15 minutes of Zumba
- 15 minutes of riding bicycle outside
- 15 minutes of hiking
- 15 minutes of any other high-intensity cardio
- 15 minutes of alternating between running and walking. Run for 1 minute, then walk for 1 minute, then run again and walk again. Repeat the cycle for 15 minutes.
- 10 sets of jog punches (45 seconds of active exercise followed by 30 seconds of rest is considered 1 set)

Advanced

Doing the exercises as described below will fulfill a 15-minute exercise commitment, even if it doesn't take 15 minutes to complete them. In fact, in most cases, you can finish them in half that time depending on your level of conditioning and how aggressive you are.

- 8 sets of plank jacks (10 jacks per set)
- 3 sets of squat jumps (10 consecutive jumps per set)
- 5 sets of mountain climbers (30 seconds of continuous exercise followed by 35 seconds of rest is considered 1 set)
- 3 sets of box jumps (10 consecutive jumps per set)
- 3 sets of tuck jumps (10 consecutive jumps per set)
- 5 sets of ice skaters (35 seconds of exercises followed by 35 seconds of rest is considered 1 set)
- 3 sets of jumping lunges (10 consecutive jumps per set)

DAY 3

Meal 1
Choose one of the following:
- 2-egg omelet with diced veggies and 3 tablespoons shredded cheese or 1 slice of cheese 3½ inches square
- 12-ounce fruit smoothie (300 calories or less; no added sugar)
- 12-ounce protein shake (300 calories or less; no added sugar). Try the Sumptuous Strawberry Shake (see recipe, page 287).

Snack
- Any item 100 calories or less

Meal 2
Choose one of the following:
- 1½ cups cabbage, lentil, tomato, or black bean soup
- Veggie and hummus sandwich on 100% whole-grain or 100% whole-wheat bread
- Chicken sandwich on 100% whole-grain or 100% whole-wheat toast with lettuce, cheese, and tomato optional and your choice of 1 tablespoon mayonnaise or 2 tablespoons mustard or dressing and a small salad
- Victorious Vegan Chili (see recipe, page 261)

Snack
- Any item 100 calories or less

Meal 3
Choose one of the following:
- Bean, vegetable, and cheese enchilada on 6-inch whole-grain tortilla

- 1½ cups poke bowl with brown rice, avocado, edamame, cucumber
- Very Vigorous Vegetable Soup (see recipe, page 266)

Snack
- Any item 100 calories or less

Exercise
Rest day

| | | | | | | | | | | | | | | | **DAY 4** | | | | | | | | | | | | | | | |

Meal 1

Choose one of the following:

- Grilled cheese sandwich on 100% whole-grain or 100% whole-wheat bread (2 slices of cheese 3½ inches square)
- 1 cup low-fat or fat-free plain Greek yogurt with ⅓ cup granola or muesli and ¼ cup berries
- Toasty Tuna Melt (see recipe, page 259)

Snack

- Any item 100 calories or less

Meal 2

Choose one of the following:

- Black bean wrap with avocados, diced tomatoes, lettuce, and brown rice on whole-grain tortilla
- Large green salad (all or any of the following: lettuce, 5 olives, 3 tablespoons shredded cheese, 5 cherry tomatoes, 2 tablespoons nuts, sliced cucumbers) with 2 tablespoons low-fat or fat-free vinaigrette-type dressing and 3 ounces sliced chicken or ½ cup beans if desired; no bacon bits and no croutons
- Creamy avocado sandwich: Spread 2 tablespoons low-fat cream cheese over 2 slices of 100% whole-grain or 100% whole-wheat bread, then cut ½ ripe avocado into slices and spread over the bread.
- Turkey sandwich on 100% whole-grain or 100% whole-wheat toast with lettuce, cheese, and tomato optional and your choice of 1 tablespoon spread like mayonnaise or 2 tablespoons mustard or dressing and a small salad
- Sprightly Watermelon Feta Salad (see recipe, page 267)

Snack

- Any item 100 calories or less

Meal 3

Choose one of the following:

- 4 servings of steamed or raw veggies with 1 cup brown rice

- 1½ cups whole-grain spaghetti with optional diced zucchini, squash, peppers, tomatoes, and/or broccoli in a marinara or lemon-wine sauce

- Tomato pesto pasta (1 cup cooked whole-wheat penne pasta with 2 tablespoons pesto and 5 halved cherry tomatoes cooked in a skillet in olive oil until soft)

Snack

- Any item 100 calories or less

Exercise

- 12,000 steps throughout the day. Use your wearable device or smartphone to keep track.

- 15 sets of stairs (up and down is considered 1 set).

| | | | | | | | | | | | | | | **DAY 5** | | | | | | | | | | | | | | | |

Meal 1

Choose one of the following:

- 12-ounce smoothie (300 calories or less; no sugar added)
- 12-ounce protein shake (300 calories or less; no sugar added). Try the Creamy Chocolate Shake (see recipe, page 288).
- 1 cup steel-cut oats with optional 1% or 2% milk, fruit, and ½ teaspoon brown sugar
- 2 scrambled eggs with diced veggies and 3 tablespoons shredded cheese or 1 slice of cheese 3½ inches square

Snack

- Any item 100 calories or less

Meal 2

Choose one of the following:

- 2 cups tomato, cucumber, onion, and black or white bean salad with 2 tablespoons balsamic vinaigrette
- Hummus chicken salad: In a bowl, combine ¾ cup shredded or diced cooked chicken and ⅓ cup hummus of your preferred flavor and spread between 2 pieces of 100% whole-grain or 100% whole-wheat bread.
- Lettuce, cheese, and tomato sandwich on 100% whole-grain or whole-wheat toast with your choice of spread
- 1½ cups soup (tomato, chicken noodle, black bean, pea, cucumber, or squash). Try the Easy Tomato Soup (see recipe, page 262).

Snack

- Any item 100 calories or less

Meal 3

Choose one of the following:

- Cauliflower and brown rice stuffed peppers (both halves of a small pepper)
- Portobello mushroom steaks: First marinate in spices and soy sauce or balsamic vinaigrette, then cook with a touch of olive oil and salt and pepper to taste.
- 6-ounce piece of baked or grilled fish with 2 servings of vegetables. Try the Honey Soy Glazed Salmon (see recipe, page 274).
- 6-ounce piece of baked or grilled chicken with 2 servings of vegetables

Snack

- Any item 100 calories or less

Exercise

30 minutes of cardio. Choose 2 of the following exercises for a total of 30 minutes:

Gym Options

- 15 minutes of walking/running on treadmill
- 15 minutes on elliptical machine
- 15 minutes on stationary bicycle
- 15 minutes of swimming laps
- 15 minutes on stair climber
- 15 minutes of spinning
- 15 minutes on rowing machine
- 20 minutes of treadmill intervals

Non-gym Options

- 8 sets of frog jumps (10 jumps per set)
- 5 sets of running high knees (35 seconds of running followed by 35 seconds of rest is considered 1 set)

- 4 sets of stationary squats (15 squats per set)
- 10 sets of butt kicks (35 seconds of exercise followed by 35 seconds of rest is considered 1 set)
- 10 sets of line hops (35 seconds of exercise followed by 35 seconds of rest is considered 1 set)
- 15 minutes of jogging outside
- 225 jump rope revolutions
- 15 minutes of brisk walking
- 15 minutes of walking up and down a staircase of at least 10 stairs; walking up and down the staircase is considered 1 set (rest between sets as needed)
- 15 minutes of Zumba
- 15 minutes of riding bicycle outside
- 15 minutes of hiking
- 15 minutes of any other high-intensity cardio
- 15 minutes of alternating between running and walking. Run for 1 minute, then walk for 1 minute, then run again and walk again. Repeat the cycle for 15 minutes.
- 10 sets of jog punches (45 seconds of active exercise followed by 30 seconds of rest is considered 1 set)

Advanced: Note that doing the exercises as described below will fulfill a 15-minute exercise commitment, even if it doesn't take 15 minutes to complete them. In fact, in most cases, you can finish them in half that time depending on your level of conditioning and how aggressive you are.

- 8 sets of plank jacks (10 jacks per set)
- 3 sets of squat jumps (10 consecutive jumps per set)
- 5 sets of mountain climbers (30 seconds of continuous exercise followed by 35 seconds of rest is considered 1 set)

FAST BURN!

- 3 sets of box jumps (10 consecutive jumps per set)
- 3 sets of tuck jumps (10 consecutive jumps per set)
- 5 sets of ice skaters (35 seconds of exercises followed by 35 seconds of rest is considered 1 set)
- 3 sets of jumping lunges (10 consecutive jumps per set)

|| | || | || | || | || | DAY 6 | | | || | || | | | | || | | | | |

Meal 1
Choose one of the following:

- 1 cup low-fat or fat-free plain Greek yogurt with ⅓ cup muesli and ¼ cup berries
- 1 slice of avocado toast on 100% whole-grain or 100% whole-wheat bread
- 12-ounce fruit smoothie (300 calories or less; no added sugar)
- 1 protein shake (300 calories or less; no added sugar)

Snack:
- Any item 100 calories or less

Meal 2
Choose one of the following:

- 1 hummus wrap (hummus, large leaf lettuce, sliced cucumbers, dill in a whole-grain flour wrap)
- Broccoli cheddar quesadilla: Place a 10-inch whole-wheat tortilla in a skillet over medium heat, spread cooked broccoli over the tortilla, top with 3 tablespoons shredded cheddar cheese and fold over. Cook on both sides until cheese melts and tortilla is golden brown.
- Large green salad (all or any: lettuce, 5 olives, 3 tablespoons shredded cheese, 5 cherry tomatoes, 2 tablespoons nuts, sliced cucumbers) with 2 tablespoons low-fat or fat-free vinaigrette-type dressing and 3 ounces sliced chicken or ½ cup beans if desired; no bacon bits and no croutons
- Smooth Lentil Soup (see recipe, page 264)

Snack
- Any item 100 calories or less

Meal 3

Choose one of the following:

- Vegetable stir-fry in olive oil with broccoli, brown rice, peppers, carrots, soy sauce, mushrooms, organic honey
- 1½ cups whole-grain spaghetti with optional diced zucchini, squash, peppers, tomatoes, and/or broccoli in a marinara or lemon-wine sauce. Try the Chickpea Pasta with Pesto (see recipe, page 276)

Snack

- Any item 100 calories or less

Exercise

Rest day

DAY 7

Meal 1

Choose one of the following:

- 1½ cups cold cereal (7 g or less sugar)
- 2-egg omelet with diced veggies and 3 tablespoons shredded cheese or 1 slice of cheese 3½ inches square
- 8-ounce yogurt parfait
- Herbed Egg-White Wraps (see recipe, page 257)

Snack

- Any item 100 calories or less

Meal 2

Choose one of the following:

- 2 slices of tomato-cheese toast on 100% whole-grain or 100% whole-wheat bread
- Bean burrito with cheese and sour cream in whole-grain flour tortilla (use black or refried beans, low sodium)
- Turkey sandwich on 100% whole-grain or 100% whole-wheat toast with lettuce, cheese, and tomato optional and your choice of 1 tablespoon spread like mayonnaise or 2 tablespoons mustard or dressing and a small salad
- Mighty Meatless Taco (see recipe, page 270)

Snack

- Any item 100 calories or less

Meal 3

Choose one of the following:

- Vegetable stir-fry in olive oil with broccoli, brown rice, peppers, carrots, soy sauce, mushrooms, organic honey
- 1½ cups non-creamy soup with a small green garden salad

- Steak salad (6 ounces thinly sliced steak over a bed of 2 cups arugula, 1 plum tomato cut into wedges, 1 sliced scallion, ⅓ cup sliced pineapple, and 1 tablespoon fresh lime juice)

Snack
- Any item 100 calories or less

Exercise
- 12,000 steps throughout the day. Use your wearable device or smartphone to keep track.
- 15 sets of stairs (up and down is considered 1 set).

Fast Forward

One of the most common questions people have when finishing a program is, "So, what's next?" In this case, the answer is simple: Carry on! One of my biggest goals with this plan was to create an independence so that you won't be on an overly structured plan forever. I wanted you to have learned a lot about food, your body, and your capacity to achieve, so that you would develop healthier behaviors and eliminate some of those bad habits that have caused you to struggle. You now have a tried and true blueprint for how you can live the rest of your life.

Once you finish the nine weeks, don't simply go back to eating all the foods you had been eating before you started the program. That also doesn't mean you can't have some fun. It's completely fine to have a good steak and French fries and even a slice of double chocolate cake (my mouth is watering just writing that!), but it's important that you add these foods back in moderation, not just in their frequency but also their quantities. Don't eat pizza four days a week or an entire family-size bag of potato chips in two days. Instead, make a list of five items you've missed the most, then every seven or ten days, add one of them back, but add it back in a small amount. The goal is to still allow yourself to eat these fun foods but to do so occasionally rather than all of the time. Seventy percent of what you eat should be tasty, but also healthful, and striking this balance will go a long way in helping you maintain weight and improve your health.

Lastly, the physical plan you just followed and this book itself can be an eternal reference guide for your nutritional and physical life. It can sit on your shelf, always accessible and never too far away, easily pulled down when you need to get yourself back on track. Just like your car needs to go to the mechanic periodically for a tune-up, the same is true of our bodies. This plan is your mechanic, available to you whenever you want, and ready to change your oil, lubricate the joints, and work out some of the glitches that are preventing you from feeling, looking, and functioning at the level you desire. You don't always have to go back and do the entire program. In fact, you can choose certain weeks that you enjoyed and that produced good results, and just follow them. You might've liked weeks 2, 4, and 9. Simply take those weeks and go back to work. You now know what it takes to win. Take the lessons learned, keep your mind focused, and be confident as you stay in the fight!

12

Fast Burn Recipes

THESE RECIPES WILL GIVE YOU CREATIVE WAYS TO ENJOY food that is healthy, yet still tasty. Like all recipes, they are just a blueprint for you to follow. You can tweak and modify according to the flavor profile that you prefer. Most of them make multiple servings, so if you're preparing food for a smaller amount of people, simply reduce the ingredients accordingly, or make as much of the recipe as you want and store the extras so you can eat them later. Most importantly, have fun with these recipes and use them as a springboard for your creative inspiration in the kitchen. You will soon learn that putting your own spin on a recipe is a lot easier and more fulfilling than you might've thought. Happy cooking and creating!

The Burner Smoothie

This smoothie is the *signature* drink of the *FAST BURN* plan. It's full of nutritious ingredients that will increase your metabolism and facilitate greater fat burn. From fiber to antioxidants and vitamins, these ingredients work together to not only make you feel full but also promote the body's ability to release energy from your fat stores. You can drink this smoothie as a meal anytime you want during the program or anywhere that calls for a shake or smoothie. You can also drink it as a snack, but make sure you only drink 8 ounces. The Burner in its full portion is meant to be a meal replacement whose potpourri of phytonutrients will always be great fuel for your body.

Serves 4
Serving size: 10 ounces

¾ cup 100% apple juice (substitute with water or milk if you want a less sweet drink)

1 teaspoon apple cider vinegar

1 teaspoon coconut oil

1 cup frozen or fresh blueberries

1 apple, peeled and cored

1 very ripe banana

½ cup baby spinach

1 tablespoon fresh lemon juice

½ cup ice cubes

Combine the ingredients in a blender, putting the liquids in first and the ice last. Blend until smooth and your desired consistency. Enjoy!

Baked Apple Heaven

Serves 4

4 large apples (Honeycrisp or Empire)

¾ cup old-fashioned rolled oats

⅓ cup pecans, chopped

¼ teaspoon grated nutmeg

1 teaspoon ground cinnamon

1½ tablespoons coconut oil, melted

1 tablespoon organic maple syrup

½ cup apple cider

1. Preheat the oven to 425°F.

2. Wash your apples under warm water and dry the skin. Using a knife or corer, core the apples, making sure to remove the entire core and pips. Keep the skin on. Grease a baking dish with cooking spray, then place the apples in the dish.

3. In a bowl, combine the oats, pecans, and spices. Then stir in the melted coconut oil and maple syrup. Mix well. Divide the oat mixture evenly among the apples, placing it in the cored-out centers. Pour the apple cider in the bottom of the baking dish, then cover with foil and bake for about 30 minutes total, basting the apples with cider every 5 to 10 minutes. Uncover the apples for the last 10 minutes, baking until fork tender. Serve warm. Enjoy!

Gramma's Old-Fashioned Scratch Pancakes

Serves 4

1½ cups all-purpose flour

3 teaspoons baking powder

1 tablespoon granulated sugar

½ teaspoon salt

1¼ cups whole milk

½ teaspoon pure vanilla extract

2 tablespoons butter, melted

1 egg

1 tablespoon vegetable oil

1. In a large bowl, sift together the flour, baking powder, sugar, and salt.

2. Make a well in the center of the dry ingredients and pour in the milk, vanilla, butter, egg and vegetable oil. Stir just until mixed and the batter is free of lumps. Let the batter rest for 5 minutes.

3. Heat a large skillet over medium-high heat. Spray with cooking oil or lightly butter. Pour about ¼ cup batter into the skillet for each pancake. Cook until golden brown on the underside and then flip. Continue cooking until both sides are brown and serve warm. Repeat with the remaining batter.

Herbed Egg-White Wraps

Serves 4

6 large egg whites

2 tablespoons low-fat milk

Salt and freshly ground black pepper

2 tablespoons chopped fresh flat-leaf parsley

1 tablespoon chopped fresh chives

6 large fresh basil leaves, finely chopped

1 tablespoon unsalted butter

Four 8-inch whole-wheat tortillas, warmed

½ cup shredded reduced-fat mozzarella cheese

1. In a medium bowl, combine the egg whites, milk, salt and pepper to taste and whisk until frothy and foamy. Add the parsley, chives, and basil and whisk again.

2. Melt the butter in a large non-stick skillet over medium-low heat, swirling to coat the pan. Add the eggs and cook, stirring slowly with a rubber spatula, until the eggs are set, about 5 minutes.

3. Divide the eggs among the tortillas and sprinkle about 3 tablespoons cheese over the eggs on each tortilla. Wrap the tortillas, folding in the ends like a burrito. Serve immediately or wrap in aluminum foil to keep warm until ready to eat. Enjoy!

Red Pepper and Scallion Scramble

Serves: 4

2 teaspoons extra-virgin olive oil

½ large red bell pepper, seeded and finely chopped

6 scallions, white and green parts separated and sliced

4 large eggs

4 large egg whites

¼ teaspoon sweet paprika

salt and freshly ground black pepper to taste

4 slices whole-grain bread, toasted

2 teaspoons whole-grain mustard

1. Heat the olive oil in a large skillet over medium heat. Add the bell pepper and scallion whites and cook until softened, 3 to 4 minutes. Reduce the heat to medium-low.

2. While they cook, whisk the eggs and egg whites together in a small bowl until combined. Add the paprika, salt and pepper to taste, and whisk to blend.

3. Pour the eggs into the skillet over the bell pepper and onions and cook until the eggs are set and scrambled, 3 to 4 minutes.

4. Spread a thin layer of mustard on each toast slice. Divide the eggs among the toasted bread slices, sprinkle the scallion greens over the top and serve.

Toasty Tuna Melt

Serves 2

One 6-ounce can tuna (try finding a brand that is pole and line caught)

2 tablespoons mayonnaise

2 tablespoons diced red onion

2 tablespoons sweet relish

1 tablespoon freshly squeezed lemon juice

Sea salt and freshly ground black pepper

4 slices 100% whole-grain or 100% whole-wheat bread

1 tablespoon butter

1 small tomato, sliced

4 slices cheddar cheese

1. Preheat the oven to 425°F.

2. Drain the tuna, then add to a medium bowl and break up with a fork into flakes. Then add the mayonnaise, onion, relish, and lemon juice. Mix together, then add some salt and pepper. Mix again.

3. Butter one side of each piece of bread. Place two slices on a baking sheet with the buttered side down. Divide the tuna salad equally and scoop it onto the bread slices. Add the sliced tomatoes on top of the tuna, then a slice of cheese on top of that. Complete the sandwich by adding the second slice, making sure the buttered side is facing up. Bake until the cheese is nicely melted, 5 to 7 minutes. Serve warm. Enjoy!

Greek Energy Bowl

Serves 4

2 tablespoons extra-virgin olive oil

Two 6-ounce boneless, skinless chicken breasts

Kosher salt and ground black pepper to taste

2 cups cooked brown rice or quinoa

1 small cucumber, cubed

1 medium avocado, thinly sliced

½ cup halved olives

1 cup halved grape tomatoes

1 cup crumbled feta cheese

½ cup balsamic vinaigrette or other clear dressing

1. In a large skillet, heat the oil over medium-high heat. Season the chicken with salt and pepper and add to the skillet. Cook until the chicken is golden brown on both sides and cooked all the way through. Once done, set aside to rest for a few minutes. Cut into thin slices.

2. Assemble the bowls: If you or your guests are not going to eat all of them, then make the others in bowls that can be refrigerated and stored for you to eat later. Scoop the brown rice or quinoa into the bowls and top with cucumber, chicken, avocado, olives, tomatoes, and feta. You can also scoop the individual ingredients into their own sections within the bowl so that they stand alone without mixing them. Once bowl is assembled, drizzle each bowl with no more than 2 tablespoons vinaigrette. Enjoy!

Victorious Vegan Chili

Serves 4

2 tablespoons extra-virgin olive oil

4 cloves garlic, minced

1 yellow onion, diced

1 red bell pepper, diced

One 14-ounce can black beans

One 14-ounce can kidney beans

Two 14-ounce cans diced or crushed tomatoes (with juices)

2 tablespoons tomato paste

1 tablespoon soy sauce

1 tablespoon ground cumin

1 teaspoon smoked paprika

¼ teaspoon cayenne powder

2 tablespoons chili powder

1 tablespoon brown sugar

1 teaspoon salt

½ teaspoon Italian seasoning

1. Add the olive oil to a large pot and heat over medium-high heat. Add the garlic, onion, and bell pepper and cook until fragrant and the onion starts to soften.

2. Add the beans, 1 cup water, the tomatoes, tomato paste, soy sauce, cumin, paprika, cayenne, chili powder, sugar, salt, and Italian seasoning and bring to a boil. Reduce to a simmer and let cook for about 1 hour.

3. If the chili is too thick, simply add water and cook a little longer. Serve warm. Enjoy!

Easy Tomato Soup

Serves 4

3 teaspoons extra-virgin olive oil

2 large carrots, peeled and diced

1 medium yellow onion, sliced

3 cloves garlic, minced

¼ cup chopped fresh basil

One 28-ounce can crushed tomatoes

½ cup tomato paste

One 14-ounce container vegetable stock

1 teaspoon dried oregano

1 tablespoon granulated sugar

½ cup light cream

2 teaspoons salt

½ teaspoon freshly ground black pepper

1. In a large pot or saucepan, heat the olive oil over medium heat. Add the carrots and onion and cook until they start to soften. Add the garlic and sauté for 2 minutes, or until fragrant. Add the basil and continue to cook until the vegetables are tender.

2. Add the tomatoes, tomato paste, vegetable stock, oregano, and sugar and bring to a boil, then let simmer over medium heat for about 20 minutes, stirring occasionally.

3. Allow the soup to cool for 5 minutes, then transfer to a blender or food processor. Blend until the desired consistency. Return the soup to the pot and add the cream, stirring it in slowly over low heat. Season with the salt and pepper. Enjoy!

Luscious Pea Soup

Serves 4

2 tablespoons butter

1 tablespoon extra-virgin olive oil

⅓ cup chopped yellow onion

2 medium celery stalks, finely chopped (1 cup)

1 clove garlic, minced

4 cups sweet peas (either frozen, fresh, or canned)

Salt

½ teaspoon freshly ground black pepper

1. Melt the butter and olive oil in a large pot over medium-high heat. Add the onion and celery and sauté until the vegetables start to soften, 7 to 8 minutes. Add the garlic and cook for about 2 minutes, until fragrant. Add the peas and 7 cups water and bring to a boil. Reduce the heat to medium and cover. Let simmer and cook, stirring often, until the peas are tender, about 5 minutes if canned and 10 minutes if frozen.

2. Add the soup in batches to a blender and puree until desired consistency. Return the soup to the pot and season with salt and pepper. Serve warm or refrigerate and serve cold. Enjoy!

Smooth Lentil Soup

Serves 4

1 tablespoon olive oil

1 large yellow onion, finely chopped

2 medium carrots, diced

3 tablespoons finely chopped celery

3 cloves garlic, minced

5 cups vegetable stock

1½ cups red lentils, rinsed and drained

1 teaspoon ground cumin

1 teaspoon curry powder

1 pinch saffron

Juice of 1 small lemon

Kosher salt and freshly cracked pepper

1. Heat the oil in a large pot over medium-high heat. Add the onion, carrots, and celery and sauté for 7 minutes, stirring occasionally. Add the garlic and sauté for 2 more minutes, until fragrant.

2. Stir in the vegetable stock, lentils, cumin, curry powder, and saffron until combined. Cook until the soup simmers, then cover and cook for 20 minutes, making sure to stir occasionally, until the lentils are completely tender.

3. Use a traditional blender or hand blender to puree the soup until the desired consistency. Return the soup to the pot and stir in the lemon juice. Season the soup with salt and pepper to taste. Serve warm. Enjoy!

Silky Butternut Squash and Apple Soup

Serves 6

2 tablespoons unsalted butter

2 cloves garlic, minced

1 small yellow onion, chopped

⅛ teaspoon ground nutmeg

1 cup cubed peeled apple (Fuji, Empire, or Gala)

2 pounds butternut squash, peeled and cubed

1 carrot, peeled and chopped

½ teaspoon sage

1 teaspoon ground cumin

3 cups low-sodium vegetable or chicken stock

½ cup fat-free evaporated milk

Salt and freshly ground black pepper

1. Add the butter to a large pot or saucepan and heat over medium-high heat. Add the garlic and onion and sauté until fragrant and the onion starts to soften, 3 to 5 minutes.

2. Sprinkle the nutmeg over the apples, then add the apples to the pot. Stir continuously for 2 minutes.

3. Add the squash, carrot, sage, cumin, and stock and bring to a boil. Cover, reduce the heat, and let simmer on low heat for about 35 minutes, until the squash is tender.

4. Discard the sage and transfer the soup to a blender or food processor. Add the milk and puree until smooth. Return the soup to the pot and simmer over very low heat for 5 minutes. Season with salt and pepper to taste. Serve warm. Enjoy!

Very Vigorous Vegetable Soup

Serves 4

4 teaspoons extra-virgin olive oil

1 small yellow onion, diced

2 medium carrots, peeled and diced

1 celery stalk, diced

Salt and freshly ground black pepper

2 cloves garlic, minced

1 teaspoon dried basil

1 pinch dried thyme

1 teaspoon oregano

2 bay leaves

3 cups vegetable broth

1 cup corn (frozen, canned, or fresh)

½ cup peas

¼ cup mushrooms

½ cup chopped red bell peppers

1 cup diced tomatoes with juices

1 cup diced sweet potatoes

1 cup fresh or frozen green beans, cut into small pieces

1 cup diced zucchini

¼ cup packed fresh parsley leaves, chopped

1. Heat the olive oil in a large saucepan. Add the onion, carrots, and celery. Season with salt and pepper and cook, stirring often, until the veggies are tender and start to brown, approximately 5 minutes.

2. Add the garlic, basil, thyme, oregano, and bay leaves as well as salt and pepper, and cook for a few minutes, stirring frequently.

3. Add the broth, corn, peas, mushrooms, peppers, tomatoes, sweet potatoes, green beans, and zucchini. Bring to a boil, then cover and reduce the heat to low. Let simmer for 15 to 20 minutes, until the vegetables are tender.

4. Remove the bay leaves and stir in the parsley. Serve warm. Enjoy!

Sprightly Watermelon Feta Salad

Serves 4

¼ cup extra-virgin olive oil

½ teaspoon sea salt

Freshly ground black pepper

½ teaspoon organic honey

2 tablespoons red wine vinegar

4 cups cubed seedless watermelon

1 cup crumbled feta cheese

½ cup thinly sliced red onion

1 cup chopped cucumber

¼ cup chopped fresh mint

1. In a small bowl, whisk together the olive oil, salt, pepper to taste, the honey, and red wine vinegar.

2. In a large bowl, combine the watermelon, feta, onion, cucumber, and mint.

3. Pour the dressing over the salad and gently toss well. Serve at room temperature. Enjoy!

Beef Burrito Bowl

Serves 4

½ teaspoon chili powder

½ teaspoon smoked paprika

½ teaspoon ground cumin

One 1-pound flank steak

2 tablespoons extra-virgin olive oil

Salt and freshly ground black pepper

2 cans black beans, drained and rinsed

2 cups frozen corn kernels

2 cups quartered cherry tomatoes

Juice of 2 limes

1 cup shredded lettuce

1 cup shredded Mexican cheese blend

½ red onion, diced

½ cup fresh cilantro

2 cups brown rice, cooked

FOR THE PICO DE GALLO (OPTIONAL)

2 cups chopped tomatoes

1 small jalapeño pepper, seeds and veins removed, diced

½ cup diced red onion

½ cup fresh cilantro, chopped

2 teaspoons fresh lime juice

Salt to taste

1. Mix the chili powder, paprika, and cumin in a small dish.

2. Cut the steak into thirds. Drizzle 1 tablespoon oil over the steak, then rub on the spice mixture evenly on both sides, then add salt and pepper to taste.

3. In a large skillet, heat the remaining oil over medium-high heat. Add the steak and sear on both sides to the desired temperature. Let rest for 5 minutes and dice into cubes or slice into thin ¼-inch strips.

4. Heat the beans in a small pot on top of the stove.

5. Heat the corn in a small pot on top of the stove or in the microwave.

6. If making the pico de gallo, combine all the ingredients in a bowl.

7. To serve, divide the rice, beans, steak, corn, shredded lettuce, tomatoes, onion, cilantro (or pico de gallo) and cheese among four bowls. Garnish with cilantro and lime juice. Serve warm. Enjoy!

Mighty Meatless Taco

Serves 4

1 cup low-sodium black beans, drained

½ teaspoon salt

1 teaspoon garlic powder

⅛ teaspoon cayenne pepper

1 teaspoon cumin

Juice from 1 lime

2 tablespoons extra-virgin olive oil

¼ cup chopped yellow onion

1 medium tomato, diced

½ cup corn, drained

¼ cup cilantro, chopped

4 whole-grain or corn tortillas

2 cups brown rice, cooked

1. Heat the black beans in a small pot.

2. In a small bowl, whisk together the salt, garlic powder, cayenne pepper, cumin, lime juice and olive oil. Set the dressing aside.

3. In a large bowl, combine the black beans, onion, tomato, corn, and cilantro. Pour the dressing over the black beans and mix well.

4. Warm the tortillas in the oven or on top of the stove. Scoop rice into the middle of a tortilla. Spoon black bean salsa over the rice. Serve warm. Enjoy.

Green Bean and Artichoke Stir-Fry

Serves: 4

8 ounces fresh green beans, trimmed and halved

2 teaspoons canola oil

One 9-ounce package frozen artichoke hearts, thawed, drained, and quartered

2 teaspoons low-sodium soy sauce

Freshly ground black pepper, to taste

4 scallions, sliced

1. Pour about ½ cup water into a large non-stick skillet (enough to cover the bottom of the pan with water). Add the beans. Bring the water to a simmer over medium-high heat. Cover the pan, and cook for 2 to 3 minutes, or until the beans are bright green.

2. Remove the pan from the heat and toss the beans, until the water is completely evaporated.

3. Add the canola oil and artichokes. Return the pan to the heat and cook, stirring frequently, until the beans begin to char, about 5 minutes.

4. Add the soy sauce and pepper and toss to coat. Remove the pan from the heat, scatter the scallions over the beans and toss to combine.

5. Transfer to a serving bowl and serve warm.

Whole Wheat Pasta with Edamame Pesto

Serves: 4

1 cup frozen shelled edamame, thawed

2 cloves garlic, chopped

¼ cup sliced almonds, toasted

¼ cup fresh flat-leaf parsley leaves

Zest of ½ lemon

⅓ cup finely grated parmesan, plus more for garnish

¼ cup extra-virgin olive oil, plus more as needed

Salt and freshly ground black pepper, to taste

1 pound whole-wheat spaghetti

1. Combine the edamame, garlic, and almonds in the bowl of a food processor and pulse until finely chopped. Add the parsley, lemon zest, parmesan, and olive oil and pulse until well combined and the edamame is very finely chopped. Transfer the pesto to a large mixing bowl and season with salt and pepper to taste.

2. Bring a large pot of water to a boil and salt it generously. Boil the pasta according to the instructions on the package. Just before draining, pour 2 or 3 tablespoons of the pasta cooking water into the bowl with the pesto and stir it to loosen.

3. Drain the pasta and transfer it to the pesto bowl and toss with tongs until well coated. Divide the pasta among four serving plates and serve with parmesan.

Tender Baked Pork Chops

Serves 4

4 bone-in pork chops about 1-inch thick

½ cup brown sugar, or 2 tablespoons organic honey (optional)

1 tablespoon sea salt

½ tablespoon ground black pepper

2 teaspoons sweet paprika

2 teaspoons roasted garlic powder

1 teaspoon ground dry mustard

½ teaspoon cayenne pepper (optional)

1 teaspoon chili powder

1 teaspoon chopped fresh thyme

2 tablespoons unsalted butter, melted

1. Preheat the oven to 425°F.

2. Place the pork chops in a large baking dish and let sit at room temperature for at least 15 minutes.

3. In a medium bowl, mix the sugar, salt, pepper, paprika, garlic powder, mustard, cayenne pepper (if using), chili powder, and thyme.

4. Coat both sides of the pork chops evenly with the melted butter. Sprinkle the dry rub evenly over both sides of the pork chops (use about 2 tablespoons per chop) and pat the spice mixture into a nice coating. Let sit for 5 minutes at room temperature.

5. Bake for about 30 minutes, until done but still tender, making sure to turn them over after 15 minutes. Cut a small slice in the middle of the pork chop to make sure it's to your desired temperature. Serve hot. Enjoy!

Honey Soy Glazed Salmon

Serves 4

4 tablespoons organic honey

4 tablespoons organic soy sauce

2 tablespoons freshly squeezed lemon juice

1 teaspoon minced ginger

2 tablespoons extra-virgin olive oil

1 clove garlic, minced

Four 6-ounce salmon steaks

Sea salt

1. In a small bowl, whisk together the honey, soy sauce, lemon juice, and ginger. Set the glaze aside.

2. Preheat the oven to 400°F.

3. In a large skillet, heat the olive oil over high heat. Add the minced garlic to the skillet, let it cook for 2 minutes, then add the salmon skin side up. Make sure the oil is hot but not smoking. Season the salmon with salt. Cook for 2 minutes, until it's nicely golden brown, then flip over and cook for another 2 minutes.

4. Take the salmon out of the skillet and place it in a baking dish. Use two-thirds of the glaze to baste both sides of each salmon steak, then place the salmon skin side down in the dish. Bake for 3 to 5 minutes. Flip the salmon with the skin side up, then baste with the remaining glaze. Put the salmon back in the oven for another 3 to 5 minutes, or until it has reached the desired temperature. Serve hot. Enjoy!

Supreme Strip Steak

Serves 4

Two 12-ounce lean, grass-fed
New York strip steaks

1 teaspoon sea salt

½ teaspoon freshly ground
black pepper

2 tablespoons extra-virgin
olive oil

2 cloves garlic, minced

2 thyme sprigs

1 tablespoon organic butter

1. Preheat the oven to 400°F.

2. Let the steaks stand for 30 minutes at room temperature.

3. Sprinkle salt and pepper evenly over both sides of the steaks.

4. Add the oil to a large cast-iron skillet and heat over medium-high. Add the steak, garlic, and thyme and cook for 2 to 3 minutes on both sides, until browned. Reduce the heat to medium-low and add the butter. Once the butter melts, baste the steaks with it and cook for another 1 minute on both sides. Transfer the skillet to the oven and roast until the steaks reach the desired temperature.

5. Transfer the steaks to cutting board and let rest for approximately 5 minutes, then slice. Serve warm. Enjoy!

Chickpea Pasta with Pesto

Serves 4

½ box (½ pound) chickpea pasta

1 teaspoon extra-virgin olive oil

1 teaspoon garlic paste

½ cup pesto

1 cup cream

½ cup organic Parmesan cheese

Freshly ground black pepper

1. Put the pasta in a large pot of water and bring to a boil, then turn the heat down to medium and let cook until al dente—about 6 minutes.

2. Heat the oil in a large saucepan over medium-high heat. Add the garlic paste, stir to separate it, and cook until fragrant, about 2 minutes. Add the pesto and cream. Stir until combined for approximately 2 minutes. Add the organic Parmesan cheese and stir frequently until the sauce is thickened. Add pepper to taste.

3. Drain the pasta well, then add it to the sauce. Stir so that everything is mixed well. Serve warm. Enjoy!

If you want to add protein to this dish, simply add diced chicken or sliced fish like salmon. You can also choose non-animal protein such as black or kidney beans.

Cheesy Chicken Quesadilla

Serves 4

2 tablespoons extra-virgin olive oil, plus more for the tortillas

Two 6-ounce boneless, skinless chicken breasts

Salt and freshly ground black pepper

4 whole-grain flour tortillas

1 cup shredded Monterey Jack cheese

½ cup shredded cheddar cheese (mild or sharp)

2 medium yellow onions, diced

½ cup salsa

1. Preheat the oven to 400°F.

2. Heat the oil in a large skillet over medium-high heat. Season the chicken with salt and pepper and add to the skillet. Cook until the chicken is golden brown on both sides and cooked all the way through. Once done, set aside to rest for a few minutes. Cut into thin slices or shred the chicken.

3. Warm up the tortillas by placing in a skillet with a little oil and slightly brown on both sides.

4. Place the tortillas on a baking sheet. Divide the cheeses, onions, and salsa among the tortillas. Load the chicken into the tortillas, then brush the edges with water and fold them over to seal the ingredients inside.

5. Bake for 5 to 8 minutes, until the cheese is nicely melted. Serve warm. Enjoy!

If you prefer to have steak, you can substitute it for the chicken.

Honey Glazed Chicken

Serves 4

4 boneless chicken thighs (for a lower-calorie option, go skinless; for more taste, keep the skin on)

Salt and freshly ground black pepper

2 teaspoons smoked paprika

1 tablespoon unsalted butter

2 cloves garlic, minced

3 tablespoons organic honey

1 tablespoon brown sugar

1 teaspoon dried thyme

1. Preheat the oven to 425°F.

2. Season the chicken with salt, pepper, and paprika on both sides.

3. Melt the butter in a large skillet over medium-high heat. Place the chicken in the skillet (skin side down if using chicken with skin) and cook until browned and crisp. Flip and cook the other side a couple of minutes less. Remove from the skillet and set aside.

4. Pour out most of the fat from the pan, but leave a couple of tablespoons. Add the garlic to the pan and stir until fragrant. Add the honey, brown sugar, and thyme to the skillet and reduce the heat to low. Return the chicken to the skillet, making sure to coat both sides with the sauce.

5. Put the skillet in the oven and bake for 20 to 25 minutes, making sure the chicken is cooked through. Serve hot. Enjoy!

Roasted Cauliflower

Serves 4

1 head of cauliflower (about 2 pounds)

4 tablespoons extra-virgin olive oil

½ teaspoon Moroccan seasoning

2 teaspoons kosher salt

MOROCCAN SEASONING (COMBINE)

1 teaspoon paprika

1 teaspoon ground ginger

1 teaspoon ground coriander

1 teaspoon ground cardamom

1 teaspoon ground cumin

½ teaspoon ground white pepper

½ teaspoon ground cinnamon

¼ teaspoon allspice

¼ teaspoon ground turmeric

¼ teaspoon cayenne pepper

1. Preheat the oven to 400°F. Cut the cauliflower into ¼-inch-thick slices and break into pieces. You should have about 8 cups.

2. In a small pan, heat 2 tablespoons oil over high heat, then add the Moroccan seasoning, cooking and stirring until fragrant (about 1 minute).

3. In a large bowl, mix the heated oil and seasoning mixture with the remaining oil. Add the salt and mix well. Add the cauliflower to the bowl, tossing well so that all pieces have a nice even coating.

4. Spread the cauliflower on a baking sheet and drizzle whatever remains of the oil mixture on top. Bake for 10 minutes, then turn the cauliflower over and bake on the second side for another 10 minutes, or until golden and tender. Serve warm or at room temperature. Enjoy!

Moroccan Sweet Potatoes

Serves 4

3 large sweet potatoes
½ teaspoon Moroccan spice mixture (see page 279)
¼ cup 100% pure maple syrup

¼ teaspoon ground cinnamon
1 tablespoon extra-virgin olive oil

1. Preheat the oven to 425°F.

2. Peel the sweet potatoes and cut into ½-inch pieces.

3. In a small bowl, whisk the Moroccan spice, syrup, cinnamon, and oil.

4. Put the sweet potatoes in a bowl and toss with three quarters of the spice mixture. Spread the sweet potato pieces on a large sheet pan, making sure to keep them as spread out as possible without any overlap of pieces. Roast for 10 minutes, then flip the sweet potatoes over and continue to roast for another 10 minutes. Drizzle the remaining spice mixture over the sweet potatoes and roast for another 10 minutes or until desired crispness. Serve warm. Enjoy!

Mango Curry Chickpeas

Serves 4

1 ripe mango

1 small handful of fresh cilantro

1-inch knob of ginger, peeled

1 cup canned tomatoes

1 tablespoon extra-virgin olive oil

1 medium yellow onion, finely diced

1 yellow bell pepper, diced

1 medium carrot, peeled and diced

1 teaspoon garam masala

¼ teaspoon cayenne pepper

¼ teaspoon ground cinnamon

1 cup coconut milk

2 cups chickpeas, drained

2 teaspoons curry powder

Salt and freshly ground black pepper

Steamed rice for serving

1. Remove the skin and pit of the mango and add the flesh to a blender, along with the cilantro and ginger. Blend well, then add the tomatoes. Blend until mostly smooth.

2. In a large skillet, heat the olive oil over medium heat, then add the onion, bell pepper, and carrot. Cook over medium heat until the vegetables are soft, about 5 minutes.

3. Add the garam marsala, cayenne, cinnamon, and coconut milk and mix well. Cook until the sauce comes to a boil, about 5 minutes.

4. Add the chickpeas, mango sauce, curry powder, and salt and black pepper to taste. Mix well and reduce the heat to medium-low. Cook until the vegetables are done to your liking and the sauce has thickened, 8 to 10 minutes. Serve over rice. Enjoy!

Knockout Brussels Sprouts

Serves 4

1 pound Brussels sprouts

3 tablespoons extra-virgin olive oil

Kosher salt and freshly ground black pepper to taste

⅓ cup balsamic vinegar

2 tablespoons organic honey (optional)

1. Preheat the oven to 425°F.

2. Trim the end from each Brussels sprout, and if the outer leaves appear dry or yellow or wilted, peel them away and discard. Cut the Brussels sprouts in half through the stem.

3. Arrange the Brussels sprouts on a rimmed baking sheet and spread out evenly. Drizzle with the olive oil and toss to coat evenly. Season with salt and pepper and toss again. Spread the Brussels sprouts cut side down in a single layer, making sure there's no overlap. Roast until the leaves are caramelized to a dark brown and crisp, 25 to 30 minutes.

4. In a small bowl, whisk the balsamic vinegar and honey (if using).

5. Drizzle the Brussels sprouts with the vinegar-honey mixture. Toss to make sure all the Brussels sprouts are evenly coated. Serve warm. Enjoy!

Crunchy Chipper Chickpeas

Serves 2

One 19-ounce can chickpeas, drained and rinsed

2 tablespoons extra-virgin olive oil

½ teaspoon kosher salt

½ teaspoon chili powder

¼ teaspoon smoked paprika

¼ teaspoon garam masala

⅛ teaspoon ground cumin

1. Preheat the oven to 400°F.

2. Pat the chickpeas with a paper towel until they are mostly dried. Let air-dry for a few minutes, then spread the chickpeas out evenly on a rimmed baking sheet. Drizzle with the oil and sprinkle with salt. Roast for 20 minutes, turning the chickpeas every 10 minutes to make sure they cook evenly, until golden and slightly darkened.

3. Meanwhile, in a small bowl, mix the chili powder, paprika, garam masala, and cumin.

4. Let the chickpeas cool for 5 minutes, then pour into a bowl. Sprinkle the spice mixture over the chickpeas and toss well. Serve warm or at room temperature. Enjoy!

Chocolate-Covered Banana Coins

Makes 20

2 medium bananas, sliced

1 cup chocolate chips (dark chocolate or milk chocolate)

½ tablespoon coconut oil

Toothpicks

1. Line a baking sheet with parchment or waxed paper.

2. Slice the bananas into ½-inch rounds. Spread the banana slices flat on the prepared baking sheet, making sure they are evenly spaced and not touching. Place in the freezer for at least 30 minutes.

3. Melt the chocolate in a double boiler on the stove, or in the microwave, until completely melted, making sure to stir occasionally. Stir the coconut oil into the chocolate.

4. Stick a toothpick into a banana slice, dip in the chocolate until completely covered, then hold up over the bowl for a few seconds to let the excess chocolate drip away. Return the banana slice to the baking sheet and repeat with the remaining banana slices. Freeze until solid, approximately 30 minutes.

5. Transfer frozen slices to an airtight freezer container and store for 2 to 3 weeks. Enjoy!

Tropical Dash Smoothie

Serves 4
Serving size: 12 ounces

1 cup pineapple chunks

1 cup mango chunks

½ cup fresh or frozen papaya chunks

½ cup low-fat or fat-free plain yogurt

2 tablespoons freshly squeezed lemon juice

½ cup milk (1% or 2% milk, soy, coconut, or unsweetened almond)

Combine all the ingredients in a blender and puree until smooth. Enjoy!

Sweet Kale-acious Smoothie

Serves 2
Serving size: 12 ounces

2 leaves green kale, stems removed

¾ cup frozen or fresh peaches

¾ cup frozen or fresh mixed berries (strawberries, blueberries, raspberries)

¾ cup apple cider or apple juice (not from concentrate)

½ teaspoon unfiltered flaxseed oil

Combine all the ingredients in a blender and puree until smooth. Enjoy!

Sumptuous Strawberry Shake

Serves 2
Serving size: 12 ounces

3 cups frozen strawberries

1 large ripe banana, peeled and sliced

1¼ cups milk (whole, 1% or 2% milk (or soy, coconut, or unsweetened almond milk)

2 tablespoons organic vanilla hemp protein powder (whey or pea protein can be substituted)

1 teaspoon organic honey

12 small ice cubes

Combine all the ingredients in a blender and puree until smooth. Enjoy!

Creamy Chocolate Shake

Serves 2
Serving size: 12 ounces

1½ cups 1% or 2% chocolate milk

1 small ripe banana, peeled and sliced

2 pitted dates

2 tablespoons fat-free chocolate yogurt

1½ tablespoons sweetened cocoa powder

10 small ice cubes

Combine all the ingredients in a blender and puree until smooth. Enjoy!

Blustery Banana Shake

Serves 2
Serving size: 12 ounces

1½ cups milk (whole, 1% or 2% milk (or soy, coconut, or unsweetened almond milk)

1 large ripe banana, peeled and sliced

2 tablespoons old-fashioned rolled oats

1 teaspoon organic honey

1 tablespoon organic vanilla hemp protein powder (whey or pea protein can be substituted)

¼ teaspoon ground cinnamon

12 small ice cubes

Combine all the ingredients in a blender and puree until smooth. Enjoy!

Sky Man's Purple Smoothie

Serves 2
Serving size: 12 ounces

¾ cup fresh or frozen blueberries

½ cup frozen purple grapes

1 cup cherries, pitted, stems removed

¼ cup fat-free plain yogurt

1 medium-size ripe banana, peeled and sliced

½ cup apple juice or cider (not from concentrate)

½ teaspoon honey

10 small ice cubes

Combine all the ingredients in a blender and purée until smooth. Enjoy!

13

Basic Training Exercises

IN THIS SECTION YOU WILL FIND SOME EXERCISES YOU CAN do to fulfill your exercise requirement in the plan. This is not an exhaustive list, but a good sampling of body weight exercises you can do to increase your heart rate and increase your muscle tone. At the end of this section are five 10-minute circuit workouts that you can also follow. Do as much as you can, and as your endurance improves, do more. The idea is simple: some exercise is better than no exercise, and do your best at whatever you try. Movement is critical not just for weight loss and fat burning, but to increase blood flow and improve brain function, stability, and mood.

BOX JUMPS

It doesn't get much simpler—a box and your legs. If you don't have a box, just use a bench in the park or on a playground. This is a tremendous exercise to increase your leg strength and tone as well as rev up your metabolism so that you burn that unwanted fat. This exercise requires more than just lower-body strength, however. Eye–foot coordination as well as good balance are required to successfully complete this maneuver. Given the heavy demand placed on your lower-extremity muscles and joints, this is not an exercise you want to do on a daily basis, but working it into your routine a couple of times a week can definitely expedite your reaching your fitness goals. Good form, with your knees bent, and a soft landing will prevent injury.

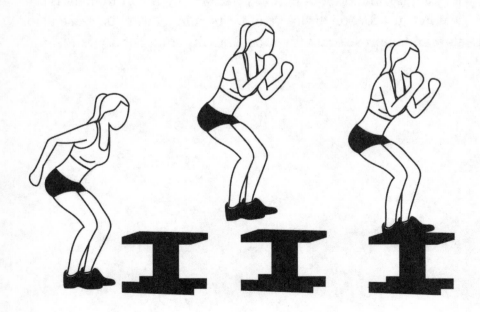

Instructions

1. Choose a box that fits your physical capabilities (2 to 3 feet high). The taller the box, the greater the physical demand to be able to jump safely atop it.

2. Stand in a relaxed position facing the box, knees slightly bent, upper body bent forward slightly at a 45-degree angle, and arms bent back against your sides.

3. In the same motion, thrust your arms forward while exploding up into the air and landing on the box with both feet in a squat position and your arms now in front to maintain your balance. Don't land on your heels; rather concentrate on keeping the weight favoring the balls of your feet.

4. Jump back off the box, return to the original position, and repeat.

BURPEES

This multi-phase exercise is a full-body exercise and is great at targeting your core, arms, chest, back, glutes, and legs. Expect a good spike in your heart rate and burn in your muscles. This exercise is most beneficial when you try to complete a certain number of burpees in a specific time. To challenge yourself as you become familiar with the exercise, increase the number of burpees you perform in that same period or increase the length of time you do the burpees.

Instructions

1. Stand with your feet spread hip-width apart and your arms resting down by your side. Put more of your weight on the front portion of your feet with your heels slightly off the ground.

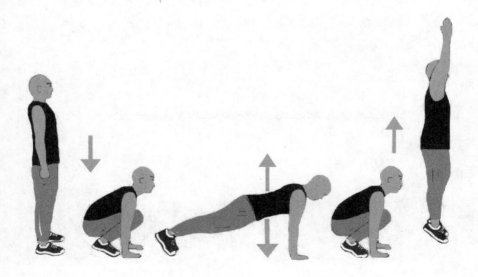

2. Lower yourself into a squat position, making sure you steady yourself by placing your hands flat on the floor in front of you.

3. Once you reach the squat position and your hands are on the floor, quickly kick your legs backward so that your body is extended into a push-up position.

4. Lower your chest to an inch above the floor just as you would if doing a push-up. Make sure you don't let your chest hit the floor.

5. In one motion, push your chest back up and pull your legs forward so that you're back in a squat position.

6. From the squat position, use your legs to push off the ground and jump as high as you can into the air, raising your arms straight overhead. Return to the starting position and repeat from step 1.

BUTT KICKS

This is meant to be a relatively simple cardiovascular exercise and is often used by runners, basketball players, and tennis players as they warm up before a game or practice. Imagine running in place but adding a new dimension of kicking your legs up behind you so that you softly tap your buttocks. You will be able to work your hamstrings and glutes and stretch your quads, which can unknowingly tighten up throughout the day.

Instructions

1. Stand erect with your arms by your sides and your feet shoulder-width apart.

2. Move forward by kicking one foot ahead and the other behind you toward your butt.

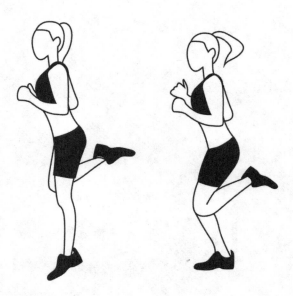

3. The hand opposite the foot touching your butt is simultaneously raised to your shoulder in a pumping motion.

4. As you lift your heels, your thighs shouldn't move. Alternate feet.

5. As you become familiar with the exercise, try to increase your speed and/or duration. If you don't completely touch your butt with your foot, don't worry. Just get it up as high as you can.

FROG JUMPS

This plyometric exercise is not for the faint of heart. It not only engages the cardiovascular and muscular systems, but in a very short period of time it can cause a spike in your metabolic demands and thus increase your caloric burn. There are two major variations of the jump, both effective at helping you meet your fitness goals.

Instructions

1. Stand in a relaxed position with your feet slightly wider than your shoulders.

2. Drop into a squat position until your thighs are parallel to the ground.

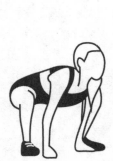 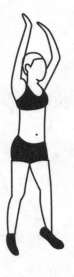 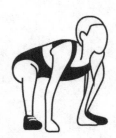

3. Keep your arms in front of you, your elbows inside your knees, your hands slightly resting on the ground.

4. Explode upward into the air while at the same time throwing your hands up.

5. Land as quietly as possible, not on your heels but on the balls of your feet.

Exercise variation: Instead of squatting and jumping in one place, you can actually perform the exercise with forward movement akin to how a frog would hop and advance at the same time. Perform the same steps above, but instead of exploding upward, make sure you're exploding upward and forward, covering as much ground as possible. Repeat this sequence for a defined number of jumps or a distance goal.

ICE SKATERS

This exercise gives you a lot of return on your investment. Imagine the speed skaters in the Olympics racing down the ice. You are going to simulate their motion, but in a static position rather than moving forward like they do. Form is important when doing this exercise, so keep your upper body slightly bent forward and your head up. Your quads will get a great burn with this exercise and your heart and lungs will also feel the rush.

Instructions

1. Start with your feet a little wider than your shoulders. Looking directly forward, keep your back straight and your knees slightly bent.

2. In one motion, take your right leg and extend it behind you toward the left side of your body so that it is farther left than your left leg; take your left hand and bend it

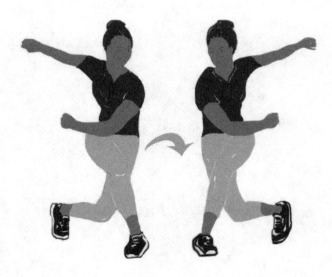

down toward the right side of your body and touch the ground.

3. Next, do the same motion, but switch sides. Bring your right leg back to its starting position and at the same time bring your left leg across behind the right side of your body; at the same time touch the ground in front of your left side with your right hand.

4. Repeat this alternating movement for the desired number of reps.

JUMPING LUNGES

This exercise takes the already demanding lunge to a higher level of difficulty, thus increasing the rewards. This is a great addition to a repertoire of full-body-weight exercises, as it doesn't require any equipment and can be done anywhere with a small amount of floor space. The benefits are diverse and tangible, engaging a spectrum of muscles, including quads, glutes, hamstrings, calves, hip flexors, hip extensors, and the core. Beyond the muscular engagement, jump lunges also work on balance and coordination, which are requirements to correctly perform this complex exercise.

Instructions

1. Start in a lunge position with one leg forward, knee bent at just above a 90-degree angle, and one leg back with the knee a few inches above the ground.

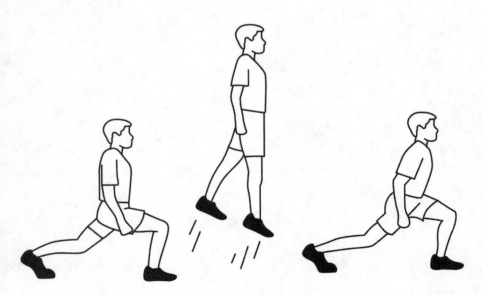

2. Hold your arms bent at the elbow at a 90-degree angle with the arm on the side of the outstretched leg also forward and the other arm back.

3. Lean slightly forward, tighten your core muscles, then quickly sink your weight down, drive both feet into the floor, and explode upward in a jump with full extension of your knees and hips so that you look like a diver jumping on a diving board.

4. While in the air and just before landing, switch positions with your feet and arms. The leg and arm that were outstretched before should now be behind you, while the other pair should be forward.

5. Controlling the landing is important, so make sure your forward knee is over your forward foot and not beyond it. Keep your hips back and make sure your knees and hips are bent to absorb all of the energy from landing. Be careful to stay flexible around your knees, making sure they aren't locked.

LINE HOPS

This is one of my favorite exercises, because it requires nothing but a line and determination. Draw a line on the ground or find a line or crack or lay down a string or rope to make the line. Jumping over the line from one side to the other is all the exercise calls for, but it can create a great physical demand when you do it for a concentrated period of time. The beauty of this exercise is that you can do the hops in a variety of forms, whether with both feet, one at a time, or simply stepping over quickly without jumping. Be prepared to work your thigh, calf, and hip muscles.

Instructions

1. Stand with both feet together on one side of a line which should be to the side of you. Both hands should

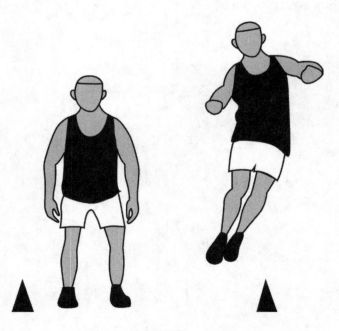

be by your side bent at a 90-degree angle as if you are about to run.

2. Slightly crouch down, then explode into the air, jumping up and laterally to clear the line with both feet at the same time and land on the other side on the balls of your feet.

3. Once you land, hop right back up and over the line to your original position.

4. Repeat this sequence, continuously jumping from one side to the other without rest.

Exercise variation: Instead of jumping with both feet, simply place one foot over the line to the other side, and once that lands, bring the other one over quickly. Pump your arms while doing this, bringing your feet back across the line in reverse order. To get your heart rate up, make sure you do this as fast as you can.

LUNGES

Lunges are a great lower extremity–strengthening exercise. When it comes to toning your legs, there aren't many exercises that can match the benefits of a lunge. There are many ways to perform this exercise, and this flexibility allows you to increase or decrease the difficulty of execution. You can do them with weights, and you can do them with jumps in between (see jumping lunges, page 302) to increase the challenge. Most important, learn the correct form, as doing this exercise improperly can cause injury.

Instructions

1. Start with your upper body straight and your shoulders held back and relaxed. Keep your chin up and head level.

2. Engage your core and step forward with one leg by lowering your hips until both knees are at a 90-degree angle—the one that is almost touching the ground and the one that is up in the air. Keep the knee that's out front

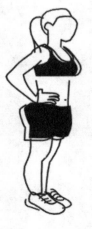
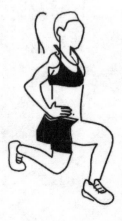

directly above your ankle without pushing it out too far. The knee closer to the ground should come close to—but not touch—the ground.

3. Once the lunge is complete, keep the weight in your heels while pushing back up to the starting position.

4. Repeat the sequence, except alternate which leg goes forward and which one goes toward the ground.

Exercise variation: When you want more of a challenge, do the same maneuver, but instead of standing back up to your original position, walk forward doing sequential lunges. This is a very advanced variation, but excellent at getting your heart rate up and increasing muscle tone.

MODIFIED GRASSHOPPER

This exercise will work your core, arms, and leg muscles. Keep your abdominal muscles tightened throughout the process for maximal contraction. The faster you go, the greater the cardiovascular workout.

Instructions

1. Start in a push-up position with hands directly underneath shoulders. Pull your right leg forward and tuck it sideways while doing so, bringing your knee up and to the left side of your body. (If doing a full grasshopper, bring your knee all the way forward so that it touches the inside of your left arm.) Make sure you tighten your core while doing this maneuver. Keep your leg off the ground throughout.

2. Return your right leg back to starting position, and then bring your left leg forward, tucking it sideways and to the right side of your body. (If doing a full grasshopper, bring your knee all the way forward so that it touches the inside of your right arm.) Keep your core tightened and legs off the ground during the maneuver. Do it faster to increase the sustained abdominal contraction and cardiovascular challenge.

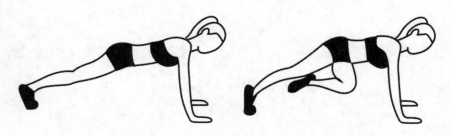

JOG PUNCHES

Jogging gets your heart rate up, burns calories, and tones your muscles. It's a perfect HIIT exercise, because you can alter your running speed according to your level of fitness or goals. To make this exercise even more beneficial and incorporate more muscle groups into the workout, punch the air while running in place. Engage your core to increase abdominal strength and toning. Make sure to breathe smoothly during the exercise and establish a rhythm.

How To

1. Stand with feet shoulder-width apart and arms in position as if you are about to jog in place.

2. Start running in place, but instead of pumping your arms forward, lift them up and punch them in the air rapidly, alternating between arms.

3. Keep pumping your arms as long as your feet are moving.

4. Perform this exercise by alternating between periods of activity and periods of rest.

MOUNTAIN CLIMBERS

This is a rigorous exercise that can pay dividends immediately and in a short period of time. This requires coordination, strength, and endurance, but when done properly, the caloric burn you achieve can be stratospheric. Start by doing small timed intervals, then increase as your endurance builds. This is a full-body exercise that will impact muscles from head to toe.

Instructions

1. Start in a push-up position, but with your hands wider than your shoulders and in front. Slightly elevate your buttocks, but not too high. Start with your left foot forward until it comes to rest on the floor under your chest. At this point your left knee and hip are bent, and your thigh is in toward your chest. Your right knee should be off the ground, with your right leg extended straight and

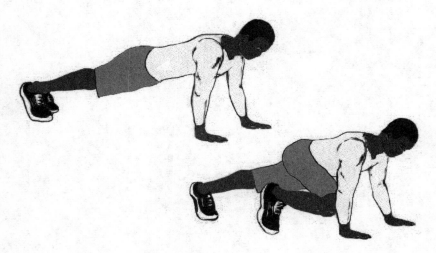

strong. Your right toes are tucked under, heel up. Contract your abdominal muscles to stabilize your spine.

2. Keep your hands firmly on the ground, and jump so that you can switch leg positions. Now your left leg is extended straight behind you and your right leg is bent underneath your chest with your right foot on the floor. Be sure to keep your abdominals engaged and shoulders strong. Do not lift your buttocks too high, as that will defeat the purpose of the exercise. Keep your head up and looking forward.

3. Repeat.

PLANK

This increasingly popular maneuver is a great addition to a regimen for anyone looking to strengthen their core and get those pronounced abdominal muscles. Doing this exercise correctly, however, is extremely important for those truly looking to maximize the gains. Perform the exercise for only the length of time that you can remain in proper form. As you become stronger, you will be able to increase the time. Don't rush. This exercise is as meditative as it is strengthening.

Instructions

1. Plant your hands on the floor, directly under your shoulders, slightly wider than shoulder-width apart. Pretend that you're about to do a push-up.

2. Press your toes into the ground and tighten your butt muscles (glutes). Make sure you don't lock or hyperextend your knees.

3. Keep your head in line with your back, and neutralize the neck and spine by focusing on a spot on the floor.

4. Hold this position for 15 seconds to start. The more comfortable and better conditioned you are, the longer you can hold the plank.

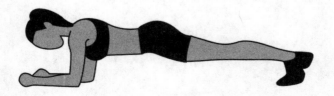

Exercise variation: To do a Forearm Plank, follow the same instructions as the regular plank, but set your forearms on the ground instead of your hands. Keep your palms flat on the ground in front of you or clasp them together—whichever is comfortable.

Exercise variation: To do a Knee Plank, rest your knees on the ground, with your forearms locked with your hands resting flat on the ground (the same position as for a regular plank). Having the knees on the ground reduces the stress in your lower back.

PLANK JACKS

This exercise is all about taking planks to the next level. Not only will you be working your core, but you will now put greater emphasis on your upper body, legs, and hip muscles. Form is extremely important for this exercise. To get the best results and to avoid injury, you must make sure you're doing the exercise correctly. Your instinct will be to lift your butt into the air so that your body is in an upside-down V formation, but this is not correct form. The exercise will be easier to complete, but you will not be maximizing the benefits.

Instructions

1. Begin in a plank position—shoulders over your wrists, back straight, body in a downward line, and feet together. You can also do the position where you rest your forearms on the ground instead of your hands.

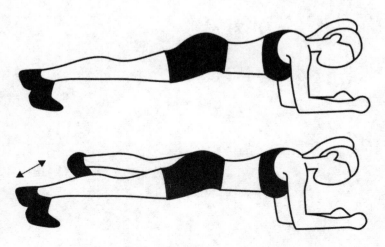

2. Imagine doing the lower portion of a jumping jack. Keep your upper body still while jumping your legs out wide, then back together. Make sure you keep your body's line intact, and don't let your buttocks pop up or your pelvis twist.

3. Decide on a specified number of jumps you want to do per set, then do at least three sets.

RUNNING HIGH KNEES

This exercise takes the marching form of high knees to a new level. The muscles that are worked remain the same, but the intensity level is increased dramatically. Instead of marching in place with your knees pumping up and your arms pumping by your side, you will now be running in place while executing the maneuver. The demand on your legs and lungs is quite high, so just a short period of exercise (30 to 45 seconds) can pay big dividends with regard to boosting metabolism and increasing muscle tone.

Instructions

1. Stand straight with your feet apart no wider than your hips. Make sure your arms are hanging down by your sides and your back is straight as you look forward.

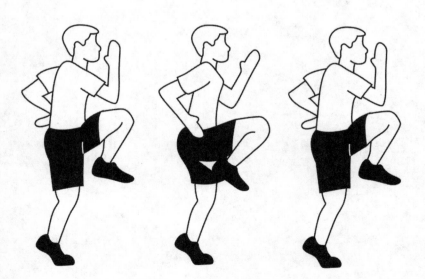

2. Jump from one foot to another as if running in place, making sure that you lift your knees as high as possible.

3. Your arms should be bent to 90 degrees with your hands clamped into fists. Pump your arms up and down in the same motion as your legs, which should be pumping up to the height of your waist.

4. Be light on your feet; make sure your heels never strike the ground, but only the balls of your feet as you continue the jumping motion for the duration of the exercise.

SQUAT JUMPS

This takes the basic squat and adds the dimension of a jump. The jumping feature will increase the intensity of muscle engagement, and the added explosiveness along with the landing are important to spike the heart rate and the fast-twitch muscles of the leg. This complex (multi-joint) exercise provides a tremendous workout in a very short period of time. Be sure to keep your knees over your ankles, not in front of them, to avoid injury.

Instructions

1. Stand up straight with your feet shoulder-width apart and hands by your side.

2. Drop into a squat position and bring your arms up to a 90-degree angle about chest high, with your hands

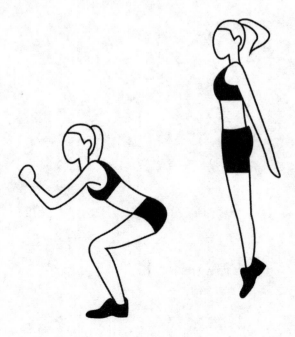

balled into fists or bent into a claw formation. Hold for 3 seconds.

3. Take a deep breath, then in one motion, bring your arms behind you like a pumping mechanism and explode into the air with your hands helping you thrust upward. Land back in a squat position when you reach the ground being careful to keep your knees over your ankles.

4. Repeat this sequence.

5. As your stamina builds, increase the number of jumps you do over a specified amount of time.

TUCK JUMPS

Tuck jumps are an explosive full-body-weight exercise that serves double duty as a cardiovascular stimulator and lower-extremity strengthener. Include this in your HIIT routine and you will find that it becomes a valuable calorie burner as it kicks your heart rate into high gear. Form is critical to the success of this exercise. Try jumping as fast as you can without compromising the form.

Instructions

1. Stand straight in a comfortable position with your knees slightly bent and core tightened.

2. Squat a little by dropping your buttocks toward the ground, then jump as high as you can.

3. Tuck your knees together and drive them up toward your chest.

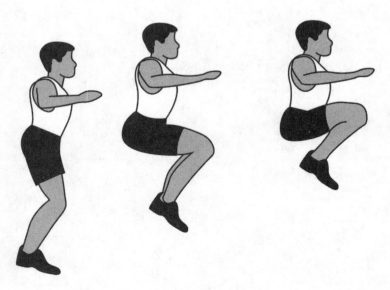

4. Land on your feet with your knees slightly bent to absorb the force as quietly as possible.

5. Repeat this sequence for a set number of jumps or for a specified amount of time.

10-MINUTE CIRCUIT WORKOUTS

Below are five circuit routines you might try for a workout. You can adjust the exercises as well as the length of time you do them and the number of sets. As you build your endurance, increase the level of difficulty or add a fourth exercise to the workout.

BREATHLESS

Ice Skaters

- 30 seconds on, 35 seconds rest = 1 set
- Complete 3 sets

Line Hops

- 30 seconds on, 35 seconds rest = 1 set
- Complete 3 sets

High Knees

- 30 seconds on, 35 seconds rest = 1 set
- Complete 3 sets

STAMINA

Mountain Climbers

- 25 seconds on, 35 seconds rest = 1 set
- Complete 3 sets

Butt Kicks

- 30 seconds on, 30 seconds rest = 1 set
- Complete 3 sets

Frog Jumps

- 30 seconds on, 30 seconds rest
- Complete 3 sets

MOXIE

Tuck Jumps

- 30 seconds on, 30 seconds rest = 1 set
- Complete 3 sets

Plank Jacks

- 40 seconds on, 30 seconds rest = 1 set
- Complete 3 sets

Lunges

- 30 seconds on, 30 seconds rest = 1 set
- Complete 3 sets

ELEVATION

Burpees

- 25 seconds on, 35 seconds rest = 1 set
- Complete 3 sets

Squat Jumps

- 25 seconds on, 35 seconds rest = 1 set
- Complete 3 sets

Jumping Lunges

- 25 seconds on, 35 seconds rest = 1 set
- Complete 3 sets

DISRUPTION

Box Jumps

- 25 seconds on, 35 seconds off
- Complete 3 sets

Modified Grasshoppers

- 30 seconds on, 30 seconds off
- Complete 3 sets

Planks

- 40 seconds on, 30 seconds off
- Complete 3 sets

Continue Your Journey to Wellness and Happiness

Regardless of how great a plan might be written, you will only get out of it what you put into it. No one wants to be on a diet forever, rather it's much more enjoyable to live, eat, and have fun. The most essential part of **FAST BURN** are all the lessons you've learned about yourself, your resilience, your strengths, and your weaknesses. You now know how to make better decisions, and while they will not always be perfect, you also know it's easy to bounce back if you stay focused, determined, and positive. You should feel confident with your new knowledge of what it takes to win, and whenever you feel like things are moving a little too much in the wrong direction, you will have **FAST BURN** right there ready to help you get back on track. You now have the power!

14

Fast Burn Snacks

S NACKS ARE A QUINTESSENTIAL COMPONENT TO A HEALTHY eating plan. They can help keep you from overindulging when you sit down to eat a meal, and they can bridge the gap between meals, keeping your hunger at bay. Snacks are instrumental, but they should not be abused. A snack is exactly that—a snack, not a meal. Unfortunately, too many people confuse the two and eat as many calories in a snack as they do a full meal. Below you will find two lists—one for 100-calorie snacks and the other for 150-calorie snacks. These lists are meant to give you ideas of the diversity of snacks you can eat that will help knock back that hunger, but also prevent you from consuming too many calories. These are not the only snacks you can eat. If you find other snacks that fit the caloric criteria, then go ahead and have them. Please note, however, that snacks that contain either protein or fiber or a combination of the two are more effective at keeping you full longer. Hopefully, the snacks below will get your creative engines turning and you will think of more options that will help fill the void.

100 Calories or Less

Fruits

- ½ small apple, sliced, with 2 teaspoons peanut butter
- ¼ cup loosely packed raisins
- 1 cup mixed berries (try raspberries, blueberries, or blackberries)
- Citrus-berry salad: 1 cup mixed berries (raspberries, strawberries, blueberries, and blackberries) tossed with 1 tablespoon freshly squeezed orange juice
- 2 medium kiwis
- ¼ avocado, smashed, on a whole-grain cracker, sprinkled with balsamic vinegar and sea salt
- Stuffed figs: 2 small dried figs stuffed with 1 tablespoon reduced-fat ricotta and sprinkled with cinnamon
- 1 cup cherries
- 30 grapes
- 1 cup strawberries
- 2 small peaches
- 3 pineapple rings in natural juices
- 2 cups watermelon chunks
- 3 dried apricots stuffed with 1 tablespoon crumbled blue cheese
- Small baked apple (about the size of a tennis ball) dusted with cinnamon
- Chocolate banana: ½ frozen banana dipped in two squares of melted dark chocolate
- 2 pineapple rounds, each ¼ inch thick, grilled or sautéed
- 5 frozen yogurt-dipped strawberries (dip strawberries in yogurt, then freeze)

- 1 medium grapefruit sprinkled with ½ teaspoon sugar, broiled if desired
- 6 dried apricots
- 4 dates
- 3 fresh figs
- ½ pound fruit salad
- 1 pomegranate
- 1 nectarine
- 3 to 4 tablespoons dried cherries
- 1 fat-free mozzarella cheese stick with ½ medium apple (about the size of a baseball), sliced with skin left on
- 1 cup fresh red raspberries with 2 tablespoons plain yogurt
- ½ cup diced cantaloupe topped with ½ cup low-fat cottage cheese

Veggies

- Kale chips: ⅔ cup raw kale (stems removed) baked with 1 teaspoon olive oil at 400°F until crisp
- ½ medium baked potato with a touch of butter or 1 tablespoon sour cream
- 1 medium red pepper, sliced, with 2 tablespoons soft goat cheese
- 10 baby carrots with 2 tablespoons hummus
- 5 cucumber slices topped with ⅓ cup cottage cheese and salt and pepper
- White bean salad: ⅓ cup white beans, a squeeze of lemon juice, ¼ cup diced tomatoes, 4 cucumber slices
- ⅓ cup wasabi peas

- ½ cucumber (seeded) stuffed with one thin slice of lean turkey and mustard or fat-free mayonnaise
- Chickpea salad: ¼ cup chickpeas with 1 tablespoon sliced scallions, a squeeze of lemon juice, and ¼ cup diced tomatoes
- 1 ounce cheddar cheese with 4 to 5 radishes
- 1 ounce cream cheese with 4 to 5 celery sticks
- 2 stalks celery
- 3 oven-baked potato wedges
- 1 large carrot, raw
- ¾ cup carrots, cooked
- 1 cup broccoli florets with 2 tablespoons hummus
- ⅔ cup sugar snap peas and 3 tablespoons hummus
- ½ cup edamame and sea salt to taste
- 1 medium cucumber
- 1 cup lettuce, drizzled with 2 tablespoons fat-free dressing
- Greek tomatoes: 1 tomato (about the size of a tennis ball) chopped and mixed with 1 tablespoon feta cheese and a squeeze of lemon juice
- Cheesy breaded tomatoes: 2 roasted plum tomatoes, sliced and topped with 2 tablespoons breadcrumbs and a sprinkle of organic Parmesan cheese
- 1 cup sliced zucchini, seasoned with salt to taste
- Grilled portobello mushroom stuffed with roast veggies and 1 teaspoon shredded low-fat cheese
- 1 cup radishes, sliced or chopped
- 1 medium ear of corn on the cob with seasoning
- 1 medium tomato with a pinch of salt
- ⅓ cup canned red kidney beans

- 1 medium tomato, sliced, with a sprinkle of feta cheese and olive oil
- 1 baked medium tomato sprinkled with 2 teaspoons organic Parmesan cheese
- Black bean salsa over 3 roasted eggplant slices
- 3 medium breadsticks with hummus
- 1 tablespoon peanuts and 2 tablespoons dried cranberries
- 1 cup grape tomatoes
- ¼ red bell pepper, sliced, ¼ cup thin carrot slices, ¼ cup guacamole
- ½ cup black beans topped with 2 tablespoons guacamole
- Stuffed tomatoes: 10 halved grape tomatoes stuffed with a mixture of ¼ cup low-fat ricotta cheese, 1 tablespoon diced black olives, and a pinch of black pepper

Nuts and Seeds

- 10 cashews
- 2 tablespoons sunflower seeds
- 17 pecans
- 2 tablespoons poppy seeds
- 2 tablespoons pumpkin seeds
- 2 tablespoons flaxseeds
- 25 peanuts, oil-roasted
- 3 tablespoons roasted unsalted soy nuts
- 12 chocolate-covered almonds
- ½ cup roasted pumpkin seeds (keep in shells)

Dairy

- ½ cup low-fat or fat-free plain Greek yogurt with a dash of cinnamon and 1 teaspoon honey

- 1 small scoop low-fat frozen yogurt
- 1 strip low-fat string cheese
- ¾ ounce sharp cheddar cheese cubes
- 4 to 6 ounces fat-free or low-fat plain Greek yogurt
- ½ cup low-fat cottage cheese with ¼ cup fresh pineapple slices

On the Go

- Leaf lettuce roll-up stuffed with a single slice of ham or beef and cabbage, carrots, or peppers
- Tropical cottage cheese: ½ cup fat-free cottage cheese with ½ cup chopped fresh mango and pineapple
- 1 hard-boiled egg with everything bagel seasoning
- 8–10 chocolate kisses
- ½ cup fat-free yogurt and ½ cup blueberries
- ½ whole-wheat English muffin topped with 1 teaspoon fruit butter
- 6-ounce glass of orange juice (try making frozen juice pops for a cooling treat)
- 2 slices of deli turkey breast
- Watermelon salad: 1 cup raw spinach with ⅔ cup diced watermelon, sprinkled with 1 tablespoon balsamic vinegar
- Strawberry salad: 1 cup raw spinach with ½ cup sliced strawberries and 1 tablespoon balsamic vinegar
- Crunchy kale salad: 1 cup kale leaves, chopped, with 1 teaspoon honey and 1 tablespoon balsamic vinegar
- Cucumber sandwich: ½ English muffin with 2 tablespoons cottage cheese and 3 slices cucumber
- Cucumber salad: 1 large cucumber, sliced, with

2 tablespoons chopped red onion and 2 tablespoons apple cider vinegar

- 1 hard-boiled egg and ½ cup sugar snap peas
- Turkey roll-ups: 4 slices smoked turkey rolled up and dipped in 2 teaspoons honey mustard
- ½ cup unsweetened applesauce with 1 slice of 100% whole-wheat toast, cut into 4 strips for dunking
- 9 to 10 black olives
- ½ cup raisin bran
- 1 cup grape tomatoes and 6 wheat crackers
- 7 saltines
- Spicy black beans: ¼ cup black beans with 1 tablespoon salsa and 1 tablespoon fat-free Greek yogurt
- ⅔ ounce dark chocolate
- Mini rice cakes with 2 tablespoons low-fat cottage cheese
- One 11½-ounce can low-sodium V8 100% vegetable juice
- ½ sheet matzo
- 20 grapes with 15 peanuts
- ⅓ cup cooked quinoa
- ¼ cup low-fat granola
- ½ cup oat cereal, toasted
- ½ cup clam chowder, preferably tomato-based
- 5 pitted dates stuffed with 5 whole almonds
- ½ cup unsweetened applesauce mixed with 10 pecan halves

Meat and Seafood

- 6 large clams
- 3 ounces cooked fresh crab
- 1½ ounces cooked Pacific halibut

- 2 ounces cooked lobster
- 10 cooked bay scallops
- 4 cooked large sea scallops
- 2 ounces cooked yellowfin tuna
- 8 small shrimp and 3 tablespoons cocktail sauce
- 2 ounces smoked salmon
- 6 oysters
- 10 cooked mussels
- 3 ounces tuna, canned in water
- ½ cup canned crab
- 3 ounces cooked cod
- 2 ounces lean roast beef

Fun

- 15 mini pretzel sticks with 2 tablespoons fat-free cream cheese
- 25 oyster crackers
- 6 saltine crackers with 2 teaspoons peanut butter
- 4 whole-wheat crackers and 2 servings fat-free cheese
- Guac and chips (5 tortilla chips and ⅓ cup guacamole)
- 1 thin brown-rice cake spread with 1 tablespoon peanut butter
- Dark chocolate and peanut butter (½-ounce dark chocolate square with 2 teaspoons organic peanut butter)
- 3 teaspoons natural peanut butter
- 1 rice cake with 1 tablespoon guacamole
- 3 crackers lightly spread with peanut butter
- About 40 goldfish crackers

- 7 animal crackers
- 3 cups air-popped popcorn
- 2 cups air-popped popcorn with 1 teaspoon butter
- 11 blue-corn tortilla chips
- 1½ cups puffed rice
- ½ cup low-fat salsa and 5 small (bite-size) tortilla chips
- 2 graham cracker squares and 1 teaspoon peanut butter, sprinkled with cinnamon
- 1 seven-grain Belgian waffle

150 Calories or Less

Fruit

- 1 medium orange, sliced and topped with 2 tablespoons chopped walnuts
- 15 frozen banana slices
- 1 medium mango
- ¾ cup halved strawberries topped with a squirt of whipped cream
- ½ cup dried apricots
- 1 medium papaya with a squeeze of lime juice on top, sprinkle of chili powder optional
- 6 dried figs
- 25 frozen red seedless grapes
- 1 cup raspberries topped with a squirt of whipped cream
- 20 medium-size cherries
- 1 large apple, sliced, sprinkled with cinnamon
- 1 medium apple, sliced, with 1 tablespoon natural peanut butter spread on the slices

- 1 medium pear and 1 cup low-fat or skim milk
- ½ avocado topped with diced tomatoes and a pinch of pepper
- 1 cup blueberries with a squirt of whipped cream

Veggies

- ¾ cup roasted cauliflower with a pinch of sea salt
- 10 baby carrots dipped in 2 tablespoons light salad dressing
- ¾ cup steamed edamame (baby soybeans in the pods)
- ½ medium avocado sprinkled with sea salt
- 1 small baked potato topped with a mixture of salsa and 1 tablespoon shredded low-fat cheddar cheese
- 1 cup sugar snap peas with 3 tablespoons hummus
- Loaded pepper slices: 1 cup red bell pepper slices topped with ¼ cup warmed black beans and 1 tablespoon guacamole
- Small baked potato topped with salsa
- 1 medium red bell pepper, sliced, with ¼ cup guacamole
- Tasty pepper: 1 sliced bell pepper, marinated in 1 tablespoon balsamic vinegar, salt, and pepper
- ½ cup roasted chickpeas
- 1 cup grape tomatoes
- 2 dill pickle spears

Nuts and Seeds

- 9 chocolate-covered almonds
- ½ cup shelled pistachios
- ½ cup roasted pumpkin seeds, lightly salted to taste
- 16 cashews

- 21 raw almonds
- 46 pistachios
- 2 medium-size nectarines

Dairy

- ½ cup low-fat cottage cheese with 1 tablespoon natural peanut butter mixed in
- 1 chocolate fudge sugar-free pudding with 5 slices strawberries and a squirt of whipped cream
- 1 slice of Swiss cheese and 8 olives
- 1½ strips of low-fat string cheese
- 2 scoops of sorbet
- 1 small chocolate pudding
- ½ cup light natural vanilla ice cream
- 1 cup yogurt parfait and 1 tablespoon granola
- ½ cup no-salt-added cottage cheese and almond butter
- 1% cottage cheese mixed with 1 tablespoon almond butter

On the Go

- 4 saltine jelly sandwiches: sugar-free jelly between 2 saltine crackers; 8 crackers in all
- Peanut butter and jelly: ½ whole-grain English muffin, 1 tablespoon peanut butter, and sugar-free jelly
- Egg salad: 2 whole eggs, ½ teaspoon low-fat mayo, and spices to taste spread on ½ toasted whole-wheat or whole-grain bagel
- 16 saltines
- Hummus and cucumbers: ½ large cucumber, chopped and combined with 2 tablespoons hummus

- Applesauce and cereal: 1 applesauce pouch and ½ cup dry cereal
- 2 hard-boiled eggs with a pinch of salt and pepper
- 2 frozen fruit bars (no sugar added)
- 10 walnut halves and 1 sliced kiwi
- Baby burrito: 6-inch corn tortilla, 2 tablespoons bean dip, and 2 tablespoons salsa
- Kiwi and oats: 1 kiwi, sliced, with ½ cup oat cereal
- ½ cup natural apple chips (no sugar or preservatives added)
- 2 tablespoons hummus spread on 4 crackers
- 1 cup grapes with 10 almonds
- Chocolate-dipped pretzels: Melt semisweet chocolate morsels in a microwave; dip 3 honey pretzel sticks in chocolate; put pretzels in freezer until chocolate sets.
- 50 goldfish crackers
- Brown rice vegetable sushi rolls, 5 pieces
- 1 cup sugar snap peas with 3 tablespoons low-fat hummus
- 1½ cups fresh fruit salad
- ¼ cup yogurt-covered raisins
- 2 stalks celery and 2 tablespoons natural peanut butter
- Watermelon treat: 1 cup diced watermelon topped with 2 tablespoons crumbled feta cheese
- 1 cup Cheerios
- 6 watermelon skewers: 1 cube watermelon, 1 small cube feta cheese, and 1 slice cucumber on each of 6 toothpicks
- 6 cucumber, cherry tomato, mozzarella ball skewers
- Mediterranean salad: 1 tomato, 1 medium cucumber,

½ diced red onion, sprinkled with 2 tablespoons low-fat feta cheese

- 1 packet of plain instant oatmeal, ½ cup fresh blueberries, sprinkle of cinnamon

Meat and Seafood

- 4 turkey slices and 1 medium apple, sliced
- 1 can water-packed tuna, drained and seasoned to taste
- 4 ounces chicken breast wrapped in lettuce and topped with dill mustard
- Turkey wrap: 2 slices of deli turkey breast, whole-grain flatbread, sliced tomatoes and cucumbers, and lettuce
- Turkey-wrapped avocado: ¼ avocado sliced into strips and wrapped in 3 ounces deli turkey meat
- Tuna salad: One 5-ounce can water-packed light tuna, 1 tablespoon low-fat mayo, and 1 diced sweet pickle

Fun

- 2 popsicles
- 1 small banana, sliced, and ½ ounce dark chocolate
- 2 ounces turkey jerky
- English muffin pizza: whole-wheat English muffin topped with 1 tablespoon tomato sauce, and 1 tablespoon organic Parmesan cheese and broiled
- 2 squares graham cracker and 8 ounces skim milk
- 4 chocolate-chip cookies, each a little larger than the size of a poker chip
- 10 baked whole-wheat pita chips and 3 tablespoons salsa
- 2 Fudgsicles

- Blueberries and sorbet: ½ cup fruit sorbet topped with ½ cup blueberries
- 1 ounce pretzels and 1 teaspoon honey mustard
- ½ blueberry muffin
- 1 cup strawberries dipped in 1 tablespoon melted semisweet chocolate chips
- 12 small baked tortilla chips and ½ cup salsa
- 7 olives stuffed with 1 tablespoon blue cheese
- 4 potstickers dipped in 2 teaspoons reduced-sodium soy sauce
- 5 crackers lightly smeared with peanut butter
- 2 cups air-popped popcorn sprinkled with 1 tablespoon organic Parmesan cheese

Index